Doctors at War

A volume in the series

The Culture and Politics of Health Care Work
edited by Suzanne Gordon and Sioban Nelson

A list of titles in this series is available at
www.cornellpress.cornell.edu.

Doctors at War

Life and Death in a Field Hospital

Mark de Rond

Foreword by Chris Hedges

ILR Press
an imprint of
Cornell University Press
Ithaca, New York

First published 2017 by Cornell University Press

Printed in the United States of America

Library of Congress Cataloging-in-Publication Data

Names: Rond, Mark de, author.
Title: Doctors at war : life and death in a field hospital / Mark de Rond ;
    foreword by Chris Hedges.
Description: Ithaca, New York : Cornell University Press, 2017. | Series: The culture
    and politics of health care work | Includes bibliographical references.
Identifiers: LCCN 2016036687 (print) | LCCN 2016037076 (ebook) | ISBN
    9781501705489 (cloth : alk. paper) | ISBN 9781501707933 (epub/mobi) |
    ISBN 9781501707940 (pdf)
Subjects: LCSH: Surgery, Military—Afghanistan. | Afghan War, 2001– —Medical
    care. | Military hospitals—Afghanistan. | Medicine, Military—Afghanistan.
Classification: LCC RD476.A3 R66 2017 (print) | LCC RD476.A3 (ebook) |
    DDC 617.9/9—dc23
LC record available at https://lccn.loc.gov/2016036687

To Magda

We're all a little weird. And life is a little weird. And when we find someone whose weirdness is compatible with ours, we join up with them and fall into mutual satisfying weirdness—and call it love.

Robert Fulghum, *True Love*

Contents

Foreword

Only those who have been to war see war. The images that reach the public, however horrific, are carefully sanitized, edited, and censored. If we truly saw war, what war does to human bodies, the long, agonizing struggle to ward off death by the severely wounded—like the soldier I watched die over six hours after having his legs blown off by a mine in the Kuwait desert—war would be so unpalatable it would be hard to wage.

Filmic and photographic images of war, even the ones that attempt to look at war unflinchingly, fail to capture what is fundamental to war's reality—a crippling fear, the awful stench, the deafening noise from explosions and the fire of automatic weapons, the zombielike exhaustion, the hallucinogenic landscape of overturned vehicles, rubble, severed and decapitated human bodies, the lifeless forms of small children, and the terrifying confusion. Combat is chaotic and confusing. So is its aftermath.

Over the two decades of war I covered as a reporter, whether in El Salvador, Iraq, or Bosnia, the ritual was always the same. The wounded, the crippled, and the dead were swiftly carted off stage. They were war's refuse. We did not see them. We did not hear them. They were doomed, like wandering spirits, to skirt the edges of our consciousness. They were ignored and, when they spoke of war's venal reality, reviled.

I went back to Sarajevo after covering the war for the *New York Times*. I found hundreds of invalids trapped in rooms in dingy apartment blocks. Many did not have wheelchairs. And, in buildings without elevators, these invalids, mostly young men, rarely left their darkened rooms. They were covered with scars from burns, blind, had lost limbs, or were paralyzed. They were cared for by elderly parents. What would happen when their parents died? Who would take them in? Where would they go? And yet I knew, perhaps, the awful answer to these questions. They would soon die. And many would die by taking their own lives. More Vietnam veterans committed suicide after the war than were killed during it. Two to three Iraqi and Afghan veterans kill themselves every day in the United States. War begins by calling for the annihilation of the others. It ends in self-annihilation.

The appeal of today's industrial warfare, or techno war, is that it distances the suffering of war's victims. Killing is impersonal. In techno war, dozens, even hundreds of people, who never see their attackers, die in an instant. Buildings and apartment blocks under artillery and air strikes disappear in seconds, trapping, burying, and crushing everyone inside. The intensity of the blast from a Hellfire missile sucks the oxygen out of the air and leaves the dead, including children, around the periphery of the blast scattered limp like rag dolls without a visible mark on their bodies. The wounds, for those who survive, result in disfiguration, brain damage, paralysis, blindness, amputation, and lifelong pain and trauma.

Mark de Rond's book tells this truth. By focusing on the physical effects of war on human bodies, it forces us to confront war's ugly reality. Just as war has become technologized, so has medicine.

Wounds that even a few years ago meant death, can now be treated, sending home men and women so hideously maimed and disfigured that the remainder of their lives is a living hell of unrelenting pain, suffering, humiliation, and terrible isolation.

The physicians and nurses who care for the human detritus of war carry their own burdens. They have seen, and held in their hands, the broken bodies that are sacrificed on the altar of war. They know war's toll. And they will carry these images, and the trauma that comes with them, for the rest of their lives.

De Rond was embedded with physicians who also cared for civilians, including children injured on the way to school, playing outside, or attending a wedding party. These children would invariably be sent back to poorly equipped hospitals or remote communities where there would be no more adequate care. At times those physicians whom de Rond wrote about had to give medical treatment to the opposing killers, those whom these wars have elevated—warlords, Shiite death squad leaders, Sunni insurgents, the Taliban, al-Qaida, ISIS. The numbness that is a consequence of war, that banishes what is tender, beautiful, and sacred, seeps into the lives of those physicians. They too will be forced to find their way back from the deathly miasma of war to return to the land of the living.

There is a massive propaganda industry, embraced by all institutions from schools to the press and churches, that seeks to deny the stark facts de Rond chronicles. This is why the British Ministry of Defense did not want the book published. De Rond shines a light on a reality we are not supposed to see. It is a reality, especially in an age of endless techno war, we must confront if we are to recover the human.

Chris Hedges
Princeton, New Jersey

By Way of Introduction

I intended to make it sound guileless and rather sweet
but you will see in it the little blades of social criticism
without which no book is worth a fart in hell.
John Steinbeck, *Journal of a Novel*

In a faraway land where the rains are dry and the trees blue and
the air bittersweet, and where ants are like dogs and birdsong is
not, there life goes for a song—everyone dies young. Safeguarding its
sandy southern perimeter was, until recently, a coalition of The Free
sandbagged in a ghetto the size of a small city. Camp Bastion was the
hub in an operation designed to secure for others the freedoms they
would have wished for themselves had they been less primitive. The
lowlands that surrounded the camp belong to a warrior people who
have walked these sands ever since Ibrahim bedded his maidservant
and sent her and her firstborn to fend for themselves. The ensuing
tiff was never laid to rest. These are Ishmael's brood.

Inside the camp was a field hospital that, while small, was said
to be the world's bloodiest, living proof of reason applied to
predicament to save daily those left limbless on account of our
cruel ingenuity. This most progressive of all wars featured sophisticated body armor and capable, rapid air evacuation, meaning

that casualties presented alive with injuries more severe than ever seen before in the living. Whether all of the most seriously injured wished to be rescued was another matter altogether, and one they no longer had any say in.

Built by the British 170 Engineer Group, the hospital started life as a tented contraption in April 2006 and doubled in size to fifty beds when converted into a more permanent structure in February 2008. It was designated a NATO hospital and operated jointly by British and American forces to provide emergency treatment for International Security Assistance Force (ISAF) troops wounded on Afghan soil. ISAF fielded Americans and Brits alongside troops from forty-nine other nations and had been established by United Nations Resolution 1386 in December 2001 to help train the Afghan National Security Forces, counter the Taliban insurgency, and help rebuild the country's crippled infrastructure.[1] Aside from treating troops, the hospital provided emergency care for injured locals, in many cases collateral damage of the war on terror, about a quarter of them children.

Those who inhabited the hospital made no claim to Operation Enduring Freedom, nor defended it.[2] Even when accounting for the effective use of helicopters and protective gear, their ability to save lives remains second to none, with survival rates for armed forces personnel in excess of 99 percent. Just short of twenty thousand casualties were admitted to the field hospital from April 2006 to July 2013—the period for which figures are publicly available—of which 96 percent survived their stay, when including enemy and noncombatants. Survival rates for Afghans once transferred into their local health care system are harder to come by but thought to be lower, as they tended to be less well protected gear-wise, and because not all may have been in the best of shape prior to injury and deteriorate more rapidly as a result.[3]

That said, the casualty numbers of the Afghanistan war still make for sober reading today: 3,407 coalition deaths were recorded as of October 2015.[4] Afghan civilian deaths are estimated at 106,000 to 170,000.[5] These numbers do not include those left with life-changing injuries on either side of the fence, nor those with psychological injuries. With its interest in veterans, the media have largely ignored the psychological impact of war on civilian populations, even as they constitute an estimated 90 percent of all war casualties, up from 5 percent in World War I, 50 percent in World War II, and 80 percent in the US war in Vietnam.[6] In fact, the concern with psychological injury was such that, in 2010, Afghanistan's Ministry of Public Health launched a five-year national mental health strategy designed to provide treatment for the estimated 42 to 66 percent of civilians suffering from post-traumatic stress disorder—PTSD—and mental illness, though it is unclear how meaningful these figures really are in a country that doesn't even know the size of its own population.[7]

When the moving vans arrived on September 22, 2014, Bastion's field hospital had developed a reputation for being the most successful trauma unit anywhere in the world, including in any prior war. Collective genius and good intentions went hand in hand with vanity and profanity, anxiety, rivalry, and profound moral turmoil. But among those who worked its wards there was tenderness too, and let us not forget camaraderie, and selflessness, and courage, and derring-do—the whole shebang, brittle perhaps, but quite without equal.

This slim volume tells their story. While it has its roots in serious scholarship, I have not dressed it up in the jargon, conceptual niceties, and conventions that are typical of academia. Those keen on a more analytical treatment of the material should have no trouble digging out my scholarly work. This particular manuscript is designed to evoke, written from the point of view of an academic given a unique opportunity to embed with a surgical team in Afghanistan and, as a precursor, to join them in pre-deployment training sessions over the preceding sixteen months. My six-week "tour of duty" was to correspond to the typical period of deployment for UK doctors. While their American counterparts will often stay put for several months, British doctors are expected to rejoin the fold of their National Health Service much sooner.

By the time I was served my joining papers, I had already spent a week observing many of those I would deploy with, in a cadaver lab at the Royal College of Surgeons, a stint I was to repeat twice more. Referred to as MOST (Military Operational Surgical Training), it was one of four components of pre-deployment training for surgeons and anesthetists. Its focus was predominantly technical, the aim that of practicing, and then perfecting, techniques for emergency medical interventions, including tracheotomies, fasciotomies, amputations, laparotomies, and thoracotomies.[8] A second required pre-deployment course, Hospex (Hospital Exercise), relied on amputees to act as battleground casualties (with the help of professional makeup artists) so as to allow for a real-time simulation of emergency medical treatment in a near-perfect replica of Camp Bastion's hospital. It focused on process rather than technique. The third and fourth pre-deployment exercises were not specific to medical staff and designed to provide fundamental training on security briefings, mine clearance, basic survival, medical procedures, and weapons handling.

Although this training helped surgical staff come to grips with the technical challenges they were likely to face, it did not also prepare them for the overwhelming feelings of senselessness, futility, and surrealism many were to experience. At no point during pre-deployment training, or during deployment, was the point of the war effort explained or offered up for discussion. While in private many of those deployed in Camp Bastion's hospital were highly critical of the war, these opinions were only ever expressed in private. Questions as to the purpose of their deployment would typically be answered with an "it's my job," leaving the matter of point or no point to politicians. After all, opening up that can of worms could erode morale, or the thing one cannot afford to put at risk when in battle.

This book has a singular aim: to try to portray the lived experience of those whose lives, in spurts, revolve around damage-control resuscitation and early surgical management in a war zone.[9] Simple though this sounds, lived experience cannot be plucked from trees and passed around like fruit; rather, it is something one approximates, using whatever empathy, imagination, and analytical skill required to bring into sharper focus the world as experienced by "the other." Prior to my deployment I had been asked to write an account of "what it is *really* like" to be a doctor at war. The argument, oft-repeated during the deployment, was that no book had ever been able to do justice to this lived experience, with the exception of the novel *MASH*. Richard Hornberger (who wrote the novel under the pseudonym Richard Hooker) had been a surgeon in the Korean War, and his fictional account is thought to have relied in no small degree on this experience. Since its publication in 1968—after a long struggle and many rejections by publishers—few, if any, books have been able to equal its knack for getting under the skin of surgical life at war. Plausible reasons for this vacuum include difficulty of access, the risk of censorship, or a preference to express the experience in a fictional manner as opposed to a factual one.

Perhaps the people featured here will one day write their own accounts of the war. Until then I hope this narrative may serve as a placeholder, allowing their world to come to life in all its hard-hitting realism: a world of banter and emotional turmoil, of the sacred and profane, of caring too little and too much, of playing God and of playing not. Like those left in their charge, the doctors and nurses found themselves at the receiving end of man's ultimate blood sport. And by God did they know it.

What you have here is pretty much what I wrote shortly after my return home. I have left the most visceral bits of it untouched, adding only the occasional reflection. I felt then, as I do still, a flurry of sharply conflicting emotions: despondency and sadness and yet also guilt for not feeling more deeply moved by suffering; a feverish desire not to fall back into a self-absorbed academic life yet an inability to think of what else to do; confusion about the human condition yet a determination to write about it. Editing the original text, I was struck by its increasing fury and, ultimately, sense of resignation. In reworking it, I have made little or no effort to cleanse it of these emotions. It seems to me that they are an intrinsic feature of it.

This short account was never intended as a truth-finding mission. I have made no attempt at verifying whether the stories people told each other during deployment are based in fact. Rather more relevant is that they were told in the first place, and that those new to the environment were socialized by means of them. They were stories that provided answers to a novice's questions: How do I get in trouble around here? What is valued and what is not? How do I get ahead? What do I need to be careful of? What gets a laugh? Who holds the chips? Who think they do? Stories and shared experiences help people orient themselves and inform their conduct, and it is these that I have tried to capture. Nor have

I made an effort to impose a narrative arc on the text. Life, after all, doesn't usually come with a story line—except in the broadest possible sense—and so why should it here? The ensuing challenge is nicely captured by Tim Kreider as he fesses up in the *New York Times*:

> My least favorite parts of my own writing, the ones that make me cringe to reread, are the parts where I catch myself trying to smush the unwieldy mess of real life into some neatly-shaped conclusion, the sort of thesis statement you were obliged to tack on to essays in high school or the Joycean epiphanies that are de rigueur in apprentice fiction—whenever, in other words, I try to sound like I know what I'm talking about. Real life, in my experience, is not rife with epiphanies, let alone lessons; what little we learn tends to come exactly too late, gets contradicted by the next blunder, or is immediately forgotten and has to be learned all over again. More and more, the only things that seem to me worth writing about are the ones I don't understand.[10]

The world isn't tidy. It is not our job to make it so. What we can do is pull up our chairs to get a little closer to the action and appreciate the messiness of it. To marshal this effort along, I have inserted vignettes, here and there, from books I was told I must read by those who were old hands at war. These vignettes have been selected principally because they express what I don't think I can do as adequately, as poignantly, or as artfully, or without putting anyone unnecessarily at risk.

This primer is relevant in that decisions as to what to feature in this book, what to omit, and what to mothball, are mine. I have sought to minimize the risk of confusion by focusing on a subset of people rather than including all and sundry. Clearly, a fifty-bed hospital features more than the two handfuls of individuals included here. I occasionally telescope time a little to allow the story to flow, effectively by pruning the most repetitive sequences. There are, for example, only so many amputations one can describe without risking the reader tuning out. The dialogue is virtually all verbatim, as recorded in my notes at the time, and all the events described here really did happen as described. Nothing has been exaggerated. Jack's trauma call was lifted from a videotaped call three years earlier. I have included it to illustrate a typical, and as it happens effective, emergency response literally word for word. By virtue of the manner in which deployments are timed, it so happened that a number of those involved in the trauma call were deployed in Bastion during my tour. So as to protect the identities of those involved, I have used pseudonyms and disguised identities. Soleski, in charge of the hospital and its staff, is a composite of three individuals. I have had to resort to using a composite for reasons I expect will become obvious. He remains a minor character in the book and, as such, does not affect the integrity of the narrative. These then are my attempts to render the manuscript legally unsafe should one or more of the authorities implicated here try to prosecute, or otherwise discipline, their staff. I have also destroyed my original field notes.

This book lays bare the workings of war surgery, or the normalcy of life that goes on even as the world around it collapses under the weight of its own resentment, ideology, and greed. It isn't, and was never intended to be, an attempt to criticize or downplay the brilliance and courage of those who feature in it. Rather it pops the hood on what is still widely considered a great success story to highlight one of the curiosities of organizational life. Why is it that in lifting the lid on a purring vehicle, one suddenly notices the mess inside it: the quarrels and frailties and petty annoyances, rivalries, excitabilities and doggedness, the coinciding of pleasure and shame? Why can the functional so often feel dysfunctional?

The narrative is based on a thorough set of field notes on observations of behavior, artifacts and conversations, on interviews, letters and poetry given to me by the staff, on reports of past deployments, and on e-mail exchanges. Even so, one must be careful not to generalize where this isn't warranted, given the scarcity of evidence. Of course it could be the case that this tour of duty was the exception and not the rule, that what unfolded was the consequence of a heady combination of personalities that hadn't been seen before and hasn't since, and that the hospital just happened to be over-resourced at the time, leaving many with more time on their hands than they knew what to do with. Based on my reading of many firsthand accounts of war, and on extensive conversations with current and former military personnel, I have good reason to doubt it.

Other than that I'm with Kurt Vonnegut: all of this crazy shit really happened, more or less.[11]

Doctors at War

1

Hawkeye

Hawkeye would occasionally play God.[1] As a general surgeon with extensive experience in treating war casualties, he was expected to make difficult decisions. Every bit as vociferous, gifted, and contemptuous as the *MASH* character whose nickname had stuck, he showed up during a weeklong surgical training course at the Royal College of Surgeons, a block or so down from the London School of Economics and Political Science (LSE).

The college had been established by royal charter in 1800; the trade guild on which it is based was founded as early as 1540. The Company of Barber-Surgeons, as this curious amalgamation was first called, decided to divorce barbers from surgeons on the insistence of the latter. These surgeons went ahead and built themselves an anatomy shop near Newgate Gaol, at the corner of Newgate Street and the Old Bailey, to give them direct access to the bodies of executed criminals. In medieval times, its keepers were apparently allowed to exact payment directly from prisoners, which, perhaps unsurprisingly, incentivized keepers to be creative in supplementing their take-home pay: they charged for entering the jail, for taking irons off, and for putting them back on. The jail was to be fertile soil for the college's cadaver labs, judiciously farmed to yield a steady flow of stiffs.

Today, the college stands in Lincoln's Inn Fields, London's largest public square and home to a tennis and netball court and a bandstand. Between it and the LSE stands George IV, a pub known colloquially as "the George," popular with surgical trainees and social scientists alike. It is here that one rinses body and mind of the residue of days spent in the college's clearly prosperous cadaver lab.

Pre-deployment training involved five days practicing on human cadavers made up to resemble recipients of the war's signature wounds: ballistic injuries to the legs, amputations, abdominal bleeding, and injuries to the chest, neck, and head. The corollary of perfecting surgical practice is a tangle of saturated human tissue: the abdomen open and packed with gauze after an emergency laparotomy; the skull exposed and brain visible through a two-square-inch window cleanly cut and designed to relieve pressure; the neck mangled after multiple attempts at placing a tracheostomy tube; the chest propped open like a clamshell; a fasciotomy exposing the tibia and calf muscle; a long piece of linen wrapped around the pelvic girdle to hold in place a fractured pelvis; the bits that fell off during dissection carefully placed in a Tupperware container. They, together with the body, will in due course be disposed of. It is nearly impossible to rid oneself of the gummy pong of formaldehyde, and the purging of it is what the George is there to facilitate.

It is here that Hawkeye and I had our first chinwag.*

---

* British term meaning "chat."

I didn't know at the time, though it would soon become clear, that if I were to be allowed to deploy to Camp Bastion, Hawkeye would be my chaperone and guardian. He talked at length about previous deployments—to Bosnia, Iraq, Afghanistan, Ireland—and time spent at sea ministering to sailors in their reproductive prime but confined to the company of men except when, occasionally, the ship would dock in one or other colorful port and all bets were off. He spoke of the games lads play, many of which have strong sexual connotations, and the diseases they'd bring back on board the vessel, and of the horrors of war, and of the terrible suffering that humans wreak on one another, oftentimes with little reason other than having been given leave to, and of his inability to understand how it is that people inflict anguish on children, whether out of malice or ideology or neglect. He talked about himself, about how he would never be promoted beyond his rank, because he refused to take on significant managerial duties if it meant sacrificing frontline work, and of his inability to keep his forthright, and occasionally politically incorrect, tongue in check. He was firm in the view that no resources be spent on Afghan casualties who have a better chance of winning the lottery than surviving their injuries. To keep them alive just because we can is, he said, heartless, seeing that they would be offloaded onto a local hospital with fewer resources, inferior pain meds, and different standards of care. Better to let them go comfortably and be done with.

Hawkeye is close to frontline troops, closer than many of his peers, and heir to the tales they bring back home. He is decisive and exceptionally skilled with the knife, happiest when elbow deep into a belly or chest where every vital organ and vessel—where life itself—resides. His patience with do-gooders wore thin long ago. He thinks they, like politicians, meddle in affairs of which they have little or no practical experience, foisting their armchair theorizing on a world they do not understand but feed on for piety or smugness or public opinion or political point scoring, and nothing would please Hawkeye more than to haul them by the hair of their neck into a busy operating theater to shove them face-first into that veritable war, the triumph of weapons designed, procured, and sanctioned on their watch.

His deportment is effective at hiding the benevolence inside. For while his peers fear or loathe him at times, or both, he cares deeply for those put in his care, and Royal Marines in particular. He would have been a marine himself were it not for a motorcycle accident that wrecked his wrist and left him unable to complete the monkey bars during a qualifying routine. At the time he was given the option of skipping the bars and taking a time penalty instead, but he refused. Everyone would forever know, he said, that he had been made an exception. Worse yet, he would know, so he opted for an ordinary Royal Navy career instead, qualified as a general surgeon, and made it his life's work to look after the Royals. Hawkeye understood the Royals, and they him.

As the George loosens its faucets and gives generously, those due to deploy get a chance to socialize, and as the alcohol does the inevitable, stories begin to flow of deployments past, of things seen or only heard about, things fair and unfair, surreal but oh so real at the same time. They might hate war, but going to war reminds them of why it is they decided on a medical career in the first place. It shows them there is life beyond their mundane civilian medical practice. It is as Chris Hedges said it was—war is what gives life meaning. Those who choke up take a hike to return a little while later to more merriment, to tales of naked generals and toilet seats and illicit sex, all the while working the night into a bond more intoxicating and affecting than any drug could deliver. For in the end it is camaraderie that wins small wars.

In the little sleep I did manage the first night, I seemed to be doing ward rounds, checking in on injured soldiers, except that in my dream the building looked far less like a hospital and more like a dormitory wing with small rooms to each side, and I entered one of these but slowly and uncomfortably, finding myself caught in a sleeping bag barely able to move, and the room being packed full of amputees not so much in as on top of beds, and one of the doctors I hadn't seen before taking me out of the room and roughly into the hallway I'd just come from, and angrily demanding of me what my business was, why I was here and with whose permission, and me trying to convince him that I was all right, that I had secured all the relevant permissions, and that he had no need to worry, but my riposte neither assertive nor effective and not helped by that ridiculous sleeping bag.

THE MOST COURSE was the first of four required pre-deployment courses and targeted specifically at surgeons and anesthetists. Next up was a Hospital Exercise (Hospex) staged in a near-perfect replica of the Role 3 hospital in Camp Bastion, but on a military base outside York, and designed to bring the entire hospital staff together. Cadavers had given way to real amputees. Even the sound of an approaching Chinook had been canned to be played while trauma teams awaited the arrival of casualties. The focus here was on process, inasmuch as MOST's focus had been on surgical and anesthetic technique. Everything was designed to happen in real time, except of course that surgical procedures couldn't, leading to a pointless scenario whereby surgeons would talk each other through whatever procedure they decided might save the day, only to be forced to stand by with little or nothing to do for as long as the procedure would ordinarily take. Little did I know then that the boredom experienced here would anticipate that in Camp Bastion, even if only on occasion, but when it hit it did so with a vengeance.

The third required pre-deployment module was also the longest in duration: a ten-day Operational Test and Evaluation Command (OPTEC) hosted at the Royal Navy base in Portsmouth and required for everyone about to deploy regardless of specialty or rank. Aside from a light-touch first-aid session, the emphasis was broadly on what to expect when dropped lock, stock, and barrel into a war zone. Practical sessions on what to do when taken hostage and how to identify land mines were a welcome diversion from lectures on Afghan language and culture.

"Why the fuck do we need to learn about Afghan culture?" Hawkeye had hissed during one of several PowerPoint presentations. A woman of Afghani origin had been keen for us to pick up some basic Pashto from an A4 crib sheet (actually she had said "crib shit," which Hawkeye thought hysterical), along with things to do and refrain from doing when interacting with locals.

"Why spend an hour and a half telling us not to show these ragheads our feet if we're going to shoot them anyway?" Hawkeye had said a little louder than I suspect he intended. And yet despite a gruff exterior Hawkeye was the only surgeon I would ever see hold the hand of Afghan boys and men worried sick about their plight, and delay procedures to make sure the interpreter was there to explain what the prognosis was and what would happen next. During one of our first ward rounds in Camp Bastion's hospital, he got visibly upset when a sick old Afghan barfed all over, and through, his ragtag beard but without also being given a bit of attention, save to be handed a disposable cardboard bowl for the residual.

"Why doesn't anyone give the poor sod some privacy?" he had asked. "Why not wheel the fucking curtain around?" Hawkeye had a knack for voicing what was on most people's mind, however insensitive or inappropriate, and his tendency to run detailed commentaries on what everyone was or should be doing and what was wrong with whatever was going on would become the bane of his compatriots. Otherwise, his magnificent pair of hands might have made him the ideal surgical colleague.

2

Reporting for Duty

The journey to Helmand was less challenging than I had been led to expect it would be. After a bit of shut-eye in a darkened waiting room at RAF Brize Norton—the UK's largest Royal Air Force station—Hawkeye and I were flushed out for our 0400 (4 a.m. in twenty-four-hour military time) flight to Helmand, wrung through security, and in characteristic hurry-up-and-wait fashion directed toward a further two linoleum antechambers, each crowded but lackluster for the late hour and the onset of memories of home.

I was just about to make my second bed of the night when we were called to board a plane from which any and every identifying mark had been removed or painted over. None of it mattered, of course, as we'd be on the inside looking out during our first leg en route to Central Asia. Officers were seated in business, foot soldiers in economy, which is where I would have ended up had it not been for Hawkeye's insistence that I needed a chaperone, and as he wasn't about to sit in cattle class, neither would I. Sleep came quickly, and before long we found ourselves on a desert landing strip. Rumor in the cabin was that we had landed in Bahrain, though this was never confirmed. After another hurry-up-and-wait four-hour layover in an improvised canteen (a "one in one out" fridge with a tall stack of water bottles beside it, a toilet block, sandy courtyard, and games room), we were fed bite-size into an army green TriStar for transport to Helmand, where we arrived just after 2100.

Hawkeye and I stepped out into the black fog, drifting with the tide toward a makeshift registration desk and, beyond that, our litter of worldly belongings now covered in fine desert sand. My two bags were lightweights in comparison with the camouflaged carryalls of Hawkeye: jeans and tees, a flack jacket and helmet, a couple of Moleskines and ballpoints, a Nikon D700 with three prime lenses, a sleeping bag, a box of breakfast bars in case we were caught out without dinner, toiletries, and a small photo album. Unlike everyone else here I carried no weapon—not allowed to— and my standard civilian-issue protective gear looked scrawny compared with Hawkeye's beefier military kinfolk.

There is nothing that quite compares to losing one's virgin- ity in a militarized zone. Everything here followed a function- before-form mantra. Yet even the functionalism of Frank Lloyd Wright always had a certain beauty about it, whereas here the lot was metal or rubber or canvas, grubby when used, camp when clean, the overriding scent a pomander of kerosene and exhaust fumes. Febland awaited our arrival. We had met several times prior to deployment and, I thought, had always hit it off. Still, my well-intentioned but tactless "How's the tour been so far?" met with a snappy "Well, what do you think?" followed by a painful silence. Escorted into a dusty four-by-four, him at the wheel, we made our way from the flight lines to the small hospital, trading the scent of kerosene for a medley altogether more familiar: of iodine, chlorine, ethanol, and isopropyl alcohol. There was little to see on the way of the four-by-two-mile poorly lit camp. What began as a tactical landing zone in Helmand in 2005 had grown into a garrisoned unit with the arrival, in 2006, of Thirty-Nine Engineer Regiment Royal Engineers, to become the largest British overseas base since the Second World War. It was named after the Hesco Bastions, the collapsible wire-mesh, heavy-duty-fabric-lined, stackable, sand-filled sacks designed to provide protection against bullets and bombs, and now caught in our headlights. They, and a series of large concrete slabs, also made for useful partitions, separating the British camp from the adjacent US Marine base Fort Leatherneck, Denmark's Camp Viking, and a small enclave for the Estonian contingent.

We pulled up into the ambulance bay—a concrete slab that separated the hospital's two clapboard divisions, admin and the mortuary on the left, trauma and the wards on the right, and used daily to hose down bloodied gurneys—heaved our gear from the back of the truck onto the floor, and wandered past reception into the hospital.

It had been a limbs-in-bins sort of day was the word upon entry. One Gurkha was still being worked on, his upper legs and buttocks ripped to sloppy twine by a large metal nut stuffed in with a home-made explosive. One of the orthopedic surgeons grabbed hold of his femur to assess extensive damage to his right bum cheek, bits of skin, flesh, and muscle left dangling spaghetti-like as he did so, the inside of the Gurkha's netherworld an angry red. Blood oozed out as fast as it was being pumped in, and yet staff seemed unruffled. A treatment plan was quickly put together and circulated. Scrub nurses dispensed and collected sterile cotton swabs, right hand for new, left for old, quickly and efficiently, counting out loud as they bundled dirty swabs into sets of five before chucking them in one of several yellow bin bags. The attending anesthetist let the surgeons know periodically how hard he had to work to keep up with the fading Gurkha. We meanwhile stood and watched, "thumbs up our arses," as Hawkeye put it. There were plenty of hands to go around, and where more is worse, the most helpful thing to do is to move along, as we did, to the Doctors' Room for a "near beer" before repairing to our bunks for a night without sleep under heavy, helicoptered skies.

By the time I returned to the hospital the next morning, late and weary for lack of sleep, the early morning casualties had already been dispatched to the ward or morgue, the youngest of the still warm only ten. Matching sets of double and triple amputees underlined the war's agonizing ambiguities: which is the crueler, to prop up Afghans with quick fixes and the sort of sophisticated analgesics not available locally for the handful of hours they'd spend in Bastion, or let them cash in on their convictions pronto and meet their Maker? Ingenuity, after all, can render death quick nowadays and pretty much pain-free. All had been Afghans this morning, peeled off the desert floor by a Dustoff* helicopter crew after 106 pounds of AGM-114 air-to-surface missile did precisely as it said on the tin. The absurdity of the situation was plain for all to see: one budget is used to save those a different budget tried to kill only moments ago, both propped up by the very same tax revenues.

Such morning mayhem soon became typical fare: most days began with a string of casualties picked off Afghan soil after 0400 morning patrols and helicoptered into Camp Bastion. And yet despite its predictability, I never did get used to this prebreakfast ritual, hitting home so poignantly and immediately the brutality of humanity at war with itself.

---

* "Dustoff," an acronym for "Dedicated unhesitating service to our fighting forces," is a call sign specific to US Army Air Ambulance units marked with a Red Cross (meaning it is explicitly designed not to engage in combat).

All that lives inside [our world] tears each other apart with teeth of all types—biting, grinding flesh, plant stalks, bones between molars, pushing the pulp greedily down the gullet with delight, incorporating its essence into one's own organization, and then excreting with foul stench and gasses the residue. Everyone reaching out to incorporate others who are edible to him . . . sharks continuing to tear and swallow while their own innards are being torn out. . . . Creation is a nightmare spectacular taking place on a planet that has been soaked for hundreds of millions of years in the blood of its creatures. The soberest conclusion that we could make about what has actually been taking place on the planet for about three billion years is that it is being turned into a vast pit of fertilizer.[1]

To see firsthand, each day, the primeval brutality and callousness of war made for a grim experience, even if not without its share of funny moments. Humor has long been known to be an effective coping response to trauma and features large in the popular hospital literature—think of Samuel Shem's *House of God* or Richard Hooker's *MASH*.[2] It is often directed at those thought to be "fair game." In ordinary hospitals these might include the obese or very old, or those suffering from preventable "lifestyle" diseases. Howard Becker and colleagues, in their landmark *Boys in White*, noted that medical students would treat certain patients with disdain because nursing them proved unrewarding and time consuming. By much the same token, cynicism and derogatory humor were typically aimed at Afghan casualties whose injuries were either self-inflicted (such as when they deliberately shot themselves in the foot) or the result of incompetence (such as when they accidentally put bullets into each other). To occasionally poke fun at Afghans might thus have served the dual purpose of distancing the self from the human misery of war, and of differentiating "us" from "them." It is very much an insider game that cannot, and never should, be played with outsiders.[3]

"Mine will be tucking into his first virgin right about now," said Fernsby, one of the orthopods, while wiping his specs on his scrubs. Orthopods, shorthand for orthopedic surgeons, are plentiful in Bastion, presumably because so too are amputations. Buster reached for his morning coffee, Hawkeye his rocks. There were plenty of mags to be had from the rhombus that doubled as a coffee table in the Doctors' Room so long as one didn't mind news that was news deployments ago and given the once-over a good many times. Colorful periodicals lugged along in duffel bags or snail-mailed in parcels offset the austerity of professional lit. Dankworth, the hospital's only tropical medicine specialist, had his dad ship him weekly tales of Fleet Street in a padded envelope, the padding a misguided reaction to what Dad imagined postal services in combat were subject to. In reality, shipping involved little more than an RAF plane and pencil pushers sniffing for alcohol, easily hidden when food coloring is mixed in with vodka and bottled as Listerine, with toothpaste and floss added to the package for believability. One wonders, has the RAF really not caught on to one of the oldest tricks in the deployment book?

Ty is American, like Buster, but an orthopedic rather than general surgeon. He got his secretary to send him his subscriptions with one instruction: to never in a million years include anything published by his co-resident and triple threat—a doc who can cut and write and has bedside manners. Another fourteen weeks and he would be out of here and back to Orange County and its chilled-out beach communities, Newport and Huntington and Laguna, where he can don shorts and sandals and grow sideburns for good measure, and where the girls are blond and tanned with suggestive tattoos on their lower backs, signposting that sweet Kodak moment en route to fourth base. Southern Cal is dope, Ty had said.

"Black Taliban pyjamas on my guy," Weegee replied. "Dead giveaway." Weegee is here hot on the heels from a twelve-month stint in a local hospital some six klicks (kilometers) removed from the birthplace of the Taliban, there as part of a crew designed to mentor local docs and nurses in the Afghan-operated, American-supplied military hospital, trying to help those he said didn't care much to be helped except if it meant accessing otherwise unaffordable equipment. He was beat and miles past pleasantries.

"Bloody well used up all of our platelets," said Hawkeye.

"There's two bags left." Fellows, a Lancashire anesthetist, is a greenhorn yet to prove his mettle and keener than most.

"Well, that's hardly good news, is it? Let's just hope none of our boys gets hurt or we're fucked," Hawkeye replied.

"*They* are," Weegee said.

"Sorry?"

"They. Just that you said *we*."

THE REALIZATION that fair-mindedness in combat need not be reciprocal and that there is such a thing as getting tied up in a lump of one's own moral making isn't lost on anyone. The mid-morning natter knew of the tension between the humanitarian treatment of victims of war and the recognition that treatment isn't always the kindest—let alone least painful—alternative, and that the Taliban may not give a hoot in any case, and so why should they?

"I bet you a million these ragheads don't give our boys that sort of treatment when they get injured," Hawkeye said. "We shoot a missile at them and they survive, and rather than finishing the job we fly in our most expensive asset and have our lads carry them two and a half miles on gurneys through the fucking heat with all their gear on their backs just to get them to the helicopter and pump them full of blood even if we all know they're going to die. Ever wonder what people back home would make of our using their blood to prop up the Taliban?"

Hawkeye, Fernsby, Buster, Dankworth, Ty, and Weegee spent the morning shooting the breeze, its being too early for DFAC* and yet having nothing else to do.

"They aren't fazed by death in the way we are," said Hawkeye. "You die doing the work of God it's like having won the fucking lottery."

"..."

"You know, don't you, that if the Taliban catch you you're fucked. Trick is to self-lubricate. It's what they tell you in training."

"Skipped that bit when my lot went through." Fellows glanced briefly at Weegee for reassurance.

"You'll bite the pillow all right," said Hawkeye. "They also told us not to feel guilty if you get a hard on while they're at it."

Out of pure hate. In and out and then in and then finish. . . . Only Homo sapiens *fucks out of hate. Only* Homo sapiens *has the developed consciousness that can make hate such a powerful aphrodisiac that there is no going back afterwards to love, sweetness, gentle caresses, cigarette smoke and soft music.*[4]

Sugared up on hard candy and pleased to have gotten Fellows in a tizzy, Hawkeye picked up where he'd left off, saying that one of the lads in his OPTEC cohort had asked if it would be okay if he finished himself off after.

"Should have heard the rest of the guys," Hawkeye said. "Took the piss right out of him. I told him not to give a monkey's about

---

* Dining facility.

what anyone else might be thinking, and that it wasn't a silly question, and that a quick flute solo would be just fine."

"Someone actually said that?"

"Sure. Can't have been more than eighteen, nineteen, and not the sharpest tool in the shed. But at least he wasn't afraid to say what he was thinking. Should be somewhere on the flight lines right now."

"I LEFT A CHOCOLATE BAR in the fridge last night and now some fucker has eaten it." An irritable Nithercott scrutinized the insides of the mini fridge through its glass door.

"My wife sent me a packet of Gucci* loose-leaf tea and that's gone as well," Southwark replied, his head hung right back so as to take in a now busily rooting Nithercott upside down. Southwark seemed unperturbed. Nithercott wasn't. Southwark is an orthopedic surgeon, Nithercott an anesthetist, and that might explain some of the difference in outlook. Orthopods don't usually take the sorts of risks that anesthetists or general surgeons do. They work on limbs, of which there are two in any case, whereas anesthetists control the physiology such that orthopods cannot even remove a tourniquet without their nod of approval. There are reasons that anesthetists talk of their job as protecting the patient from the surgeon, even if partly in jest. Anesthetists and general surgeons—known as gassers and slashers—have more in common with each other than either of them with orthopods or plastics.

"You might want to ask Jock about that one. He was all happy about having found a small teapot the other day and has been using it ever since."

---

* Military slang for anything bought to replace an issued piece of equipment.

Jock, "the plastic," is shameless and irreverent but in a playful sort of way, having had more human anguish burned onto his retinas than most of those here, except Hawkeye. Both are exceptional cutters. Whereas Hawkeye likes big holes, Jock, true to his discipline, prefers to keep them small. But as mostly corrective cosmetic surgery is carried out in hospitals back home, Jock has ended up spending the majority of his time working on hands and faces, picking out bits of shrapnel and, if he really must, an eye.

If one were to divvy up people into dogs and birds going by facial features, then Hawkeye's a dog. So are Jock and Fernsby. Ty, Southwark, and Dankworth are birds, their features finer, pointier, as are Bomber's and Doo Rag's.

Doo Rag is Puerto Rican and the youngest among the five general surgeons. With youth comes ambition, and Hawkeye suspected him of trying to wriggle himself into every surgical procedure just so he can add another entry into his surgical logbook. Hawkeye's beef with Bomber was similar in that Bomber is highly experienced in trauma surgery and unambiguously ambitious, one of the youngest ever to have been put in charge of a large trauma center back in Britain, and with eyes set on bigger prizes yet.

Hawkeye told Bomber of a buddy of his who, after two tours of Afghanistan, feels unworthy of wearing his green beret and cannot get it up with his missus because he remembers his best mate getting shot in the head because he couldn't be arsed to raise the height of the Hesco compound wall despite having been asked to do so the previous day, and now his mate's dead and his dick is limp and his life shit.

My roommate, Brook, was three weeks into his first tour and spent. Early this morning, as was often the case, Brook's pager summoned him to hospital for the arrival of yet another casualty of the dawn patrol. He slipped on his still-buttoned-up shirt like a sweater, crumpled its tails under his belt, and laced up his combat boots. As I heard the Chinook planting itself onto the desert floor, Brook stole into the ink outside where a fire crew was already busily shifting human cargo onto a gurney and into a specially modified Defender for its short journey to the hospital. Eighteen minutes later and Brook was back in his cotton-and-feathers pothole. "Gunshot wound to the head," he mumbled, "DOA," and sunk face-first into his pillow in search of anything but war.

Man has places in his heart which do not yet exist, and into them enters suffering in order that they may have existence.[5]

The Operation Minimize alert sounded minutes after Brook hit the bed, and in doing so, identified the fatality's nationality. Every dead Briton cranked into gear a set of bullhorns dispersed through the camp like a connect-the-dots. With it all forms of communication with the outside world are shut down instantly in an effort to prevent families back home from finding out via Facebook or otherwise before they can be visited by two people from the Ministry of Defence, there to give the news no one wants to receive or, for that matter, give.

As I walked into the hospital post-breakfast, the doctors were busily working on an Afghan shot through the spine two days ago and now paralyzed. Not satisfied with shattering three vertebrae, the bullet had churned his gut to chowder for good measure. He hadn't a prayer of surviving, or so one of the docs said. Bomber, having opened him up sternum to pubis and packed him to the rim with sterile swabs, begged to disagree. Problem was that if these were left in too long the patient risked turning septic, and if they were taken out, he risked bleeding to death with nothing left to press against his torn veins and arteries.

"We all know the score," Hawkeye said.

"Difficulty is that he is right now sitting up in bed talking," Bomber replied.

"Well, he won't be for much longer. He's septic as fuck."

"Anyone have any ideas on what we want to do about him?"

"He'll either die here or on the operating table, and as far as I'm concerned," said Hawkeye, "the operating table is more traumatic so best avoided."

"Problem is we've got to get him out of ICU before he infects everyone else," Southwark said.

"Why don't Doo Rag and I take him back into theater? If we can get him repacked and he survives, fine, he'll go straight to the ward," Bomber offered.

"And if he doesn't?" asked Hawkeye.

"Then at least we'll have given it our best shot. Either way he is not heading back to ICU."

The Afghan was swiftly whisked away from his visitor—who, hand on heart, bowed ever so slightly—then drugged up to the eyeballs by Cold Feet, a lanky, small-shouldered, large-footed anesthesiologist, who kept checking his anesthetic preps: a milky-white Propofol to induce sleep, Fentanyl to numb the pain. As Bomber and Doo Rag began the disagreeable job of plucking rancid swabs from the belly, Cold Feet worked himself up into a frenzy about plummeting blood oxygen levels, wondering out loud whether they could please stop the procedure and take him back to ICU even as Hawkeye quickly reminded him that this was precisely what they decided not to do, whatever the circumstance.

"He's not going to make it," said Cold Feet.

"We know," Bomber replied.

"So why not sew him back up and let nature take its course?" Hawkeye volunteered.

"Our gent's approaching room temperature. Anyone have a better idea?" Bomber said.

Doo Rag shook his head.

Hawkeye, never one to hesitate, said no.

Cold Feet, looking like a monkey fucking a kidney, pleaded the fifth.

And so Bomber asked for sutures and sowed the belly back up.

"Another one bites the dust," Fernsby, who had been looking in on the procedure, told Southwark back in the Doctors' Room, spinning make-believe revolvers into make-believe hip holsters.

3

Camp Bastion

Camp Bastion, before its handover in late 2014, covered eight square miles of desert in southwestern Afghanistan and served as the coalition's logistical hub in Helmand. Some six hundred aircraft flew in and out of it every day. Never short of ambition, former British prime minister Tony Blair designated it an extraordinary piece of desert where the fate of world security was sure to be decided.[1]

Its fifty-bed hospital featured an ordinary and intensive care ward, a six-bed resuscitation bay (or emergency department), referred to as "resus," a four-theater (or bed) operating room, GP and dentist practices, and a pharmacy. Its administrative wing, across the ambulance bay, held various offices as well as one morgue for the Americans and another for everyone else. Adjacent to the morgues stood a small chapel. Having begun its operations inside a large canvas tent—which remains pitched in case of emergencies—the hospital, over time, had grown into a concrete-block-and-mortar structure with the sorts of amenities one might expect from any modern facility, including two CT scanners, mobile X-ray equipment, and a fully functioning blood lab, all conveniently located within yards of one another.

In addition to handling battlefield casualties, the hospital provided useful services for troops with non-battle-related maladies: tooth extractions, appendectomies, treatments for unusual or uncomfortable growths, chronic back pain, broken bones; a merry pageant of the dead, dying, and suicidal, the sick and the sorry.

The nurses, operating department professionals (ODPs), and operating room staff lived a stone's throw away from the hospital in an enclave of their own, in eight-bed pods that divided off canvas corridors symmetrically. Khaki covers hid elaborately constructed Wendy houses inside, composed of bedsheets, flags, and towels strung together with bits of nylon. Sleeping bags like slumbering dogs lay on camping beds or stuffed inside duvet covers. Damp towels hung peg-less from coated washing lines, as did a canvas dongle with pockets for soap and undies.

Several of the pods featured a white sheet at the far end to provide cinematic entertainment at the end of a long day. Admission prices never exceeded a smile and six-pack of fat man's Coke,* though spicy chicken wings and pepperoni pizza were a definite plus. Others contained comfy chairs, collapsible and cheaply made but solid enough for late-night chinwags. The cots were plain but comfortable, the linen passed on from prior generations and yours to wash and sign over to your replacement in due course. Despite cool air pumped in through textile piping, it was often too hot to crack one off, and so one idled away the hours.

Everything in Bastion was bought and sold using American dollars. Change came in the shape of paper coins, all about an inch in diameter, and varying in colors depending on value. These could be traded for soda pop, food, candy, coffee, toiletries, and knickknackery in a small market square that featured a Pizza Hut–Kentucky

---

* Military slang for Classic Coke.

Fried Chicken combo operating out of an old shipping container. There was also a coffee shop, games room, and a NAAFI.* A bit farther down were a couple of "tourist shops" where locals displayed their trinkets. Higher-ticket items, electronics, and Americana were sold in a PX† in the adjacent Fort Leatherneck, less than a klick away.

Leatherneck belonged to the US Marine Corps. Its two most popular venues by far were the PX and canteen, the former open to everyone, the latter only to American personnel. The PX offered many more choices than did the NAAFI in stocking multiple brands of shampoo, toothpaste, deodorant, and other such essentials, lads' mags, American foodstuffs, knives, laptops, slippers, bicycles, headphones, first-aid kits, and electric razors. Turning left out the back door of the Doctors' Room and into the hot wind outside, one bore left after the first junction and followed a sandy trail alongside a Hesco wall for about ten minutes, and then, when the Hesco ended, a quick right into a ramshackle but amply stocked shop. The canteen was a little farther away but worth the extra few paces. The only way for non-Americans to get in was to fake identity, passing ID cards from a host marine down the line and signing in with a phony name. It was easily done.

Once inside, one got to harvest the war menu. Gone were the C-rations of old and in were hamburgers and chicken breasts, pizzas and corndogs, potato chips, tacos, burritos and fajitas, salads, soup, Louisiana hot sauce, ranch dressing, fresh fruit, Quaker oatmeal, Jell-O, Ben and Jerry's, milkshakes, fizzy drinks, Starbucks, Pop Tarts, Hershey's, Lucky Charms, Jelly Belly jelly beans, A&W

---

* Navy, Army and Air Force Institutes, or shorthand for a shop offering basic groceries.

† Post exchange, a common name for a type of retail store operating on US military installations worldwide.

Cream Soda and Root Beer, year-round pumpkin pie, Oreos, Reese's Pieces, chocolate chip cookies, fries with BBQ sauce or ketchup or tartar sauce, ice cream topped up with chocolate sauce or marshmallows, coffee as espresso, Americano, cappuccino, or latte, all thanks to the realization that morale might well be one of America's fiercest weapons and, in the scheme of things, also one of the cheapest.

Bastion's fifty-bed field hospital had its very own launderette: a sorry marriage of canvas, plywood, and corrugated sheeting. But it worked. It is here that staff members dropped off scrubs, soiled linens, pj's, and towels in muslin fishnet bags to have all life boiled out of them. Doctors preferred it for its speed over their accommodation's alternative and took to dropping off their personal kit, again in netted bags but with a name tag or bit of colored ribbon tying off the top end. One dropped them on a trolley, signed over power of attorney to the lads, and Bob was your uncle. Drop-offs were welcome day and night, as were pick-ups, watched over by young men occasionally seen petting two to a sofa with a third looking on, but up and about when caught out by a late-night visitor looking for something clean to wear. Muslin leftovers from past deployments had accumulated on the bottom ledge of a three-shelf rack, their owners long since gone, too tired in the end or too affected by their deployment to want to lug their relics home. The hospital never closed and neither did the laundry or, for that matter, the morgue or incinerator. It was a different story for the DFAC, where if you turned up after closing time you'd forgone your right to dinner and would have to make do on biscuits or tinned foodstuffs instead.

Hitting the sack in Bastion meant one of two things, depending on one's rank. Tier Two accommodation looked very like trailer homes stacked two floors high and featured bedrooms and ablutions along a laminated, character-free corridor. It was reserved for officers: slashers and gassers, physicians and intensive care specialists, radiologists and emergency doctors. They were a more luxurious alternative to the eight-bed tented pods occupied by nurses and ODPs, even if those were far more social. Just yesterday, health and safety had ordered the removal of all fridges, cabinets, books, and kettles from the hallway, thinking these might be obstructions in case of an evacuation. In doing so, however, they created a quite different, and not insignificant, obstacle: by ridding the cabins of all remnants of social life they also stripped them of the possibility for any form of socialization. True, there may be picnic tables outside designed for that purpose, but these were conspicuously empty except late at night when the temperature finally allowed for it.

Hawkeye did not take long to move out of Tier Two and into the eight-bunk canvas pods where, he said, the ablutions were more plentiful and less honking, where the wastewater wasn't tepid and actually drained, and man-stink didn't hang in the air like gummy fog. He bunked up with three primary care physicians. Four spare beds were occupied on and off for the odd night by those waiting for their return flight to Britain. He kept me a spare bed, he said, in case I changed my mind (which I did, three weeks in). While air-conditioned, the tented pods were many degrees warmer and stuffier. To this the solution was simple: sleep naked and trust your body to work its merry way from atop the sleeping bag to inside it as the night drove the temperature down. Unless you rose with the dawn patrol, you'd wake up dank at sunrise as the cool night had given way to the firestorm that is Afghanistan's summer.

Mosquitoes weren't ever a big deal. There wasn't a swamp within miles, and it was unlikely that the odd stray would carry malaria, and so screw the antimalarials. But the ants were big, and there were many of them, forever in a great hurry.

On the wooden patio outside the Doctors' Room stood a makeshift mast. On it were nailed handwritten signs pointing out distances to Tokyo (4,165 miles), Diego Garcia (2,720), Pyongyang (3,985), and various other destinations. Outside the patio were the Hesco defense barriers and beyond them a dirt road and more Hesco and more dirt and ultimately the flight lines (or airport) and more Hesco and the wasteland beyond. Where we thought the wild things were.

THE DOCTORS' ROOM looked a jumble: recycled furniture, long-out-of-date broadsheets, utensils, mugs, cups, and plates, none identical, a hot pad and transformer, a PC, rumors of porn on the hard drive, a telly and games console, a DVD player, three feet of DVDs, spine-cracked paperbacks, thumbed copies of *Top Gear*, *FHM*, the *Lancet*, *Homes & Gardens*, the *Week*, *Marie Claire*, the *Economist*, *Good Housekeeping*, *Hello*, *Men's Health*, *Esquire*, *Cycling*, *Cosmopolitan*, *Nuts*, *Heat*, *National Geographic*, *Country Living*, *GQ*, a couple of plastic desk chairs (one without its metal frame and bolted to an upside-down soda-pop crate), an assortment of pens and paper, a small desk, a screwdriver, winegums, strong mints, instant and filter coffee, a pack of milk raided daily from the ward, white disposable cups, sugar cubes, spilled sugar, a mini-fridge, PG tea, near beer, bottled water, tinned olives, tinned snails, tinned mushrooms, gefilte fish, flour, linoleum, a veneer back-door and outside it a cruel furnace and, improbably, a small sun-flower and tomato patch (testament to Ty's determination to make something, anything, grow in these desolate sands), some greeting cards stuck to the wall, a child's drawing of a Christmas tree and a handwritten GOB LOVES YOU next to it, a now-defunct roster, an unfinished model of a fighter jet suspended from the ceiling by fishing wire and bits of Blu-Tack, newspaper clippings, a Pirelli calendar, and a map of Afghanistan. It may have been a dreary old sack, but it was theirs.

"BASTION WILL BE BRILLIANT," Hawkeye had said prior to deployment: there'd be no booze and plenty of exercise to be had, and boy could he do with losing ten pounds. The camp was equipped with an air-conditioned gym and several smaller tents set up for the same purpose but without the luxury of machine-cooled air. Most tents had no more than a few treadmills, three or so Concept II rowing machines, and free weights. The largest and coolest of them all, even if nauseatingly warm by ordinary standards, was easily the most popular for those keen to trim their bodies. That being the case, Hawkeye much preferred the intimacy of a tented gym close to his sleeping pod. When he did muster up the courage to wake at 0500 (anytime later and it became impossible to breathe while exercising), he'd spend forty-five minutes on the treadmill—ten minutes of running followed by five of walking—topped off by two half-liter bottles of lukewarm water. The bottled water, drawn from Bastion's own freshwater well, stood on pallets in the relentless sun. Cool water required either a fridge or a predawn rise, the former meaning a trip to the hospital, the latter an unappealing prospect for those on call twenty-four seven.

As the weeks passed, trips to the gym became less frequent, as did those to DFAC. If Hawkeye couldn't drop pounds by sheer exercise he would do so, he said, by not eating. Problem was that he kept snacking from a basket of goodies in the Doctors' Room, which sat on a shelf next to the fridge and was refilled almost daily from packages received from family and friends back home. This he supplemented with tinned olives, sausage, sardines, meatballs, snails, soup, and whatever else he managed to root out from the amply supplied, multipurpose storage cabinet. The only other surgeon who would snack as much, or nearly as much, was Jock.

In the hospital, each day began and ended with a meeting of department chiefs and included many of the surgeons. It was here that patients were discussed on an individual basis and life-or-death decisions made. One such decision involved a local policeman, who had become a more or less permanent fixture on the agenda. He was referred to as a "lifer." His prognosis changed with every passing day, and the docs could not make up their minds whether to transit him into a local hospital, as was protocol, or to keep him for further treatment until such time as it would be safe to transfer him. He arrived with a belly split open by a big-caliber bullet but with a sufficiently good outlook for the docs to want to hang on to him. Keeping him here gave him the best possible chance of recovery, provided he didn't succumb to septicemia. Were he to go where the locals go, Kandahar or Lashkar Gah, he would almost certainly die. Why some Afghans got the benefit of doubt and others didn't would remain a mystery to me, though I expect it might have had something to do with the availability of beds and expectation of recovery. The problem was that he had turned septic and delirious, calling upon Allah in regular intervals to the disquiet of the soldiers and children sharing the ward.

Hawkeye and Febland meanwhile had been diverted to a British infantryman, one of three casualties of the early morning patrol. All had severe injuries to their arms and legs, and, in the case of one, his perineum. Given its proximity to anus and genitalia and the network of vessels in the pelvic cavity, the perineum, when badly wounded, can quickly become infectious and tricky to manage. Bleeding is a particular problem, as applying direct pressure to the wound is unlikely to be effective, or indeed straightforward, given its location. Thus the emergency laparotomy: a long incision using a fat blade from ribcage to pubis, followed by a cautery pen, sealing small blood vessels as it slices alongside them, along the fat underneath and the white sheath of fascia between the abdominal muscles to cleanly open up the belly and clamp off the blood supply from the inside. Invasive but effective in hemorrhage control, even if linked with high morbidity and likely to make one a hell of a lot sicker, though by that point the issue of choice is to all intents and purposes moot.

4

A Reason to Live

Having been in Bastion for over a week, I had only just managed a decent night's sleep. I genuinely cannot recall catching any sleep during my first week, though I must have, remembering only a clammy restiveness, shifting from side to side but unable to kip for the sound of helicopters and the excess adrenaline coursing impatiently through my veins.

Today got off to a busy start, and by the late afternoon the pressure had still not let up. Three of the four operating beds, or theaters, had been in use for most of the day. Theater 2 has three orthopedic surgeons debriding a popliteal fossa,* hoping to shunt the vessel in the knee pit as a temporary measure prior to repair. In Theater 3, Hawkeye and a colleague were working up a sweat over a leg that had been cold for four hours already, with little or no blood supply and no detectable pulse. The colleague had made a stab at a femoral vein graft, which didn't take, and so opted for harvesting what might well have been the only viable vein left in the leg, though if this were to fail as well, there'd be little hope for the limb to survive. Not that Hawkeye blamed him,

---

* A shallow depression at the back of the knee joint.

even if he himself would have harvested a vein from the other leg instead, or used a shunt.*

"You can't be too hard on others in these crappy conditions," Hawkeye told me. Frankly, his surgical colleague looked beat, staring unhappily at the leg that would have been his swan song. He had been operating for forty-one consecutive days, the last seven of which he said had consisted mostly of chucking dead or dying limbs in bins. Homemade explosives left few options other than lopping off the dying bits and dropping them in one of several buttercup-yellow buckets destined for the incinerator. He felt shattered, he said, the misery and moral ambiguities of the war having desiccated whatever gusto he brought to it six weeks ago, too tired to feel compassion, and yet he wouldn't think of asking for help.

Hawkeye let him plod on.

Dankworth, meanwhile, spent the afternoon outside, sunbathing, military spec shades, book, and water bottle within arm's length and unruffled by the heat. It wasn't as if he wasn't on call. It's just that as the only physician, and with no infectious cases whatsoever to look after, there'd been fuck-all for him to do, as Ty put it.

ON OUR WAY to breakfast the next morning, the indirect fire (IDF) alarm sparked a right racket. Given Bastion's size, it was always a bit of a lottery as to where mortars might land, and priorities being what they were, everyone ducked for cover and remained either flat on the desert floor or behind one of a legion of Hesco sacks or concrete walls. In the operating theater meanwhile, the surgical staff were hugging the linoleum and would need to rescrub after

---

* A long tube with a non-return valve to allow blood (or other fluids) to move from one part of the body to another.

the all clear. Though not as regular an occurrence as it once was, mortars and rockets fired from pickups still found their way into the camp every so often.

"Is that all you got?" Sloppy Joe thundered at the top of his voice as if the perpetrators were within hearing distance. "Is that all you got, you fucking losers?" He wiped the desert dust from his fatigues.

Sloppy Joe is a man of convictions, in the mold of a six-foot-four-inch Rodin, and proud of his home turf Alabama.

> *"My mother told me I'd regret coming over here. She said I'd get my ass in a crack like this and praying wouldn't help because any God that permitted this war wasn't gonna be much interested in the fate of my skinny little prick."*
> *"Your mother always talk so dirty?"*[1]

A devotee of W., Joe will happily flaunt his chauvinism regardless of circumstance or social context. Yet he is generous to a fault, keen to please, and good for a laugh, provided one took him no more seriously than he did himself. Back in Jefferson County, he runs emergency room shifts and is plenty used to triaging blunt trauma, strokes, heart attacks, kidney stones, and the odd gunshot wound (GSW) but nothing like the big open blast wounds that have become the signature injury of Afghanistan's summers.

Last night a badly injured farmer, in Joe's care, opted for a code brown. The casualty had arrived by Pedro, a similar setup to the medical emergency response team (MERT) that operates out of a Chinook, but in this case American-staffed and using the smaller Pave Hawk helicopter. Sloppy Joe, on Hawkeye's invitation, had grabbed the Afghan by the ankles and pulled them up to eyeball height, and as Hawkeye examined the lacerations behind the upper legs, he got rather more than he bargained for. Sloppy Joe retched while Hawkeye smirked, grabbing a fistful of gauze as he did so to catch and dispatch the feculence.

The excitement was fun while it lasted for those looking on, with the remainder of the morning eerily quiet. There were a couple of old wounds to close up but little coming in casualty-wise. Dankworth put on an episode of *The In-Betweeners* while Buster doled out godsends from a gray muslin postal sack. Food items automatically became communal property and were laid out on the coffee table or stuffed in a large Tupperware right next to the micro-fridge for future use. Hawkeye had been slipped a bag of sweet chili peanuts by his wife, while Fernsby received a homemade ginger cake. Fellows got a drawing by his son, Southwark some new loose-leaf Earl Grey, Jock a couple of packets of winegums, Dankworth a week's worth of cutouts of the *Times* crossword. All except the puzzles were handed over, remarked on, picked at, turned upside down, endorsed, and passed down the daisy chain.

SAVED BY THE BELL. Lunch at the DFAC was followed by live sports coverage and reruns of *M.A.S.H.*, before morphing into an altogether more interesting evening. Two casualties had been dropped off by helicopter, the elder of whom—possibly in his late forties, though it can be hard to tell with locals—was badly inebriated, his face in tatters. Word was that he had been involved in a hit-and-run collision. Neither driver nor pedestrian had been tuned in to the perils of drinking and driving in close proximity, and one of them ended up the worse for wear. The driver had buggered off, quite possibly oblivious to the difference between hitting rock and bone, and leaving nearby troops to call in a nine-liner* instead.

The man was verbally abusive, or so the interpreter explained, a little flushed, and fought off any attempt to help him or hold him down. He badly needed to go into theater for emergency surgery but didn't pass the Woolworths test,† and, given the level of his intoxication, was wrapped in gauze before being ordered onto the ward to sleep it off. He'd hopefully be able to tell the difference between a hangover and head injury by the time he woke up the next morning.

The other casualty was a thirteen-year-old who had sustained shrapnel wounds from an improvised explosive. Ball bearings penetrated the skin behind his ear and his arm, with shrapnel having entered his neck, buttocks, and hand.

"I hope the Taliban are proud of themselves," Jock spat as he readied himself to scrub. A much older man, the boy's chaperone, doted over him as, all of a sudden, the boy broke out in song, his voice pitch-perfect, the melody unknown to anyone save for his elder. It didn't bear thinking that he might be a fun boy in the pay of his chieftains, his age and singsong raising the odds, though he could just as well be a boy tenderly cared for by his father or uncle or grandfather. Hard to tell. Sadly, and difficult to get one's head around, Afghan officers, police and military included, were known

---

* A request for a medical evacuation (often by helicopter), listing location, radio frequency, and call sign, number of casualties by precedence, special equipment required, security at the pickup site, method of marking the pickup site, patient nationality and status, and the presence of any nuclear, biological, or chemical contamination.

† This is British anesthetic slang meaning that if one can imagine a patient shopping at Woolworths, a now-defunct retail chain, she or he is considered stable enough to be given a general anesthetic.

to have catamites—colloquially known as "bacha bazi" or "danc-
ing boys"—to service them.[2]

The men involved in this practice were said to have "a toothache
problem," a euphemism for a habit of sexually abusing kids. A surgeon with extensive experience in Afghanistan told me some time
after my return home about a fifteen-year-old mentally challenged
Afghan boy who had been raped so often and so viciously that his
sphincters were destroyed. He came in with a major rectal prolapse,
with six inches of ruined rectum poking out.

Sexual relations between adult males may be punishable by death,
but sex between adult men and pre-pubescent boys appeared to be
viewed quite differently. The documentary maker Ben Anderson
filmed a police chief saying that boys came of their own accord
and liked "giving their asses at night." He said that sexual abuse by
his soldiers was one of war's necessities: "If my commanders don't
fuck these boys, who will they fuck? Their own grandmothers?"[3]

He seemed amused.

Even if intimacy is reserved for marriage, this hardly protects
those most vulnerable. The surgeon went on to tell me about a
twelve-year-old girl, brought in by her new husband rather as one
might return a defective toy, who couldn't stop bleeding after their
matrimonial first night. Her vagina had been torn to shreds, and
so he sewed it up as best he could, but, as he said, henceforth she
was damaged goods.

One gets used to the fact that there are no real facts except the
ones looking back at you from a gurney. Once the boy was put
to sleep, Hawkeye focused on prying out bits of metal from his
head and buttocks while Southwark concentrated on the arm and
hand. The buttocks and head were fortunately in better shape than
the arm and hand, and so Hawkeye thinned out to do his e-mail,
before retiring bored stiff to his bunk, wishing to beat the bishop.

I, meanwhile, sat down to write to a distant colleague and friend:

From: Rond Dr M. E. J. de
To: Bud Popsugar
Subject:

Bud

Arrived safe and well in Bastion: a big dot in a bowl of sand. I have only been here for a few days and already recoil at the thought of having to stay here for another two months. The injuries are truly horrific. The people are generally friendly even if they seem unsure as to who I am or what I am here to do. Alas, that'll take time.

By the way, I took my girls to the beach the day before my departure. We had decided to take them out of school. While there, my twelve-year-old caught me reading Don Winslow's *Savages*. You'll recall that you strongly recommended the book to me. I ordered it, and it arrived a few weeks ago.

"Mum, guess what daddy is reading?" she shouted excitedly and turned around to look at my wife.

Before I knew it, she had yanked the book out of my hands and handed it to my wife. Both read from the top of page 267:

> Lado crawls into bed.
> To give the wife a little.
> What she needs, a good stiff dick.

Why are you reading this stuff? My wife said. A colleague recommended it to me, I said, and then in an attempt to redeem myself, "he's dying." And so we spent the next five minutes on the topic of your pancreatic cancer.

THE FOLLOWING MORNING brought yet another postal sack, and the usual assortment of goodies got to do the rounds. Hawkeye, Fernsby, Southwark, Fellows, and Bomber pounced on a parcel of home-sewn surgical hats, courtesy of a kind soul back home with lots of time on her hands. All were variously bright and colorful. Hawkeye was first out with a bubblegum number. Southwark opted for a black one with yellow thunderbolts. Fernsby's was blue with red lobsters. Turquoise polka dots adorned Fellows's dark blue, and Japanese calligraphy Bomber's, while Ty chose a Piet Mondrian knockoff. Within minutes the package was picked to the bones and the docs lined up for an all-smiles snap in an otherwise empty operating theater.

The proverbial hit the fan at 1650 with a steady but persistent drip of casualties. A US marine bilateral amputee never so much as made it to Camp Bastion before kicking the bucket. A second explosion took out three Brits, two of whom were fortunate to escape with minor frags. The third wasn't so lucky and has been booked on a medevac flight back to Britain tonight. Their gurneys meanwhile were taken outside for hosing off, the congealed blood watered down in a single elongated puddle that, with gravity's pull, made its way down the concrete slab and toward the small chapel and the dry desert soil surrounding it. Sand is a wonderful absorbent.

No sooner were the first lot dispatched than another handful arrived to take their place. Five of the gravest sat out the hot Helmand night in the morgue. Come two in the morning, Hawkeye, Southwark, Fernsby, and Jerrycan, a newly arrived American female orthopod, were still up to their elbows in injured Taliban. A male nurse stood idly by. "Hurry up. Movie night tonight!" read his disposable green apron in black sharpie, written several hours prior, the frivolity and silliness of it now a little misplaced.

FINDING IT DIFFICULT to find sleep that night, my thoughts turned to our pre-deployment training when, on one of our first nights in Portsmouth, Hawkeye and a few young sailors opted for a night off ship and on the town. Portsmouth has plenty to offer where night-life is concerned, pubs to begin with and then nightclubs. The first few pints went down like a dream, as did the nachos, chicken wings, chips, king prawns, onion rings, salsa and sour cream, washed down by lager. From there, and elsewhere, we moved to more spirited stuff, things like Ardbeg and Hendrick's, Sambuca and Blue Curaçao and Malibu, no rhyme or reason whatsoever to their sequencing. The more colorful were served in a vase with straws, like potato shoots, poking out, and each of us out-sucking the others for fear of losing out. The lowest common denominator rapidly became the occasion for many a joke, the conspicuous exception being our media ops bore who insisted we head back, and wasn't tomorrow an early start anyway?

One of the boys complained about being too narrow, and Hawkeye said a circumcision would solve his problem, but better have a look at it first, and no sooner had the sailor buggered off to the loo than he returned with a snapshot of his todger. Might need to take another look tomorrow morning, Hawkeye said, as he returned the phone, but it would be no biggie to pencil the procedure in his surgical roster and so why not sink another of those nice red cocktails as more were on order.

One of the younger soldiers meanwhile had asked a girl if she wanted to fuck, just like that, utterly unselfconscious and with-out shame, repeating himself twice over for the disco music, and then she said no, sorry pal, that's not going to happen. His two friends meanwhile had left the club en route to Southsea to find themselves a hooker, failed to score, spent their wages in a casino instead, and got to bed at four.

You talk to the broad for a few minutes in some social situation, pref-erably over a drink, and you say, "Honey, let's go somewhere and tear off a piece." Either she says OK, or she takes off like a candy-assed baboon. The big plus of this method is that you either score fast or lose fast, and if you lose you can go on to the next blossom without further waste of time, effort and good booze.[4]

The very first casualty of today's morning patrol was a case of "green on blue."* An Afghan whom the casualty had trained along-side of for weeks had crossed over to the other side, gone mad, or both, and fired a round straight into the soldier's belly. Bomber, as lead surgeon, grabbed the bull by the horns and opened the belly with a long sternum-to-pubis incision. Doo Rag assisted. Once done and dusted, Bomber packed the belly and wrapped the torso in sticky yellow plastic for easy opening. Draining tubes were pot-ted in sterile receptacles, allowing liquid traffic to commute in two directions via drips and infusion pumps and big-bore hypodermic needles.

Hawkeye, meanwhile, was told to stand down, as his desig-nated casualty had died en route. Dropping the odd blasphemy, he headed for the Doctors' Room and his portal to the world of e-mail, Facebook, and hard candy.

THE SCENT OF freshly fried Sunday morning breakfast pancakes hung in the long hospital corridor that stretched from reception to primary care. It was from this main artery that wards and labs and theaters grew. The waft was pleasant and heady and able to briefly subvert the usual narcotic of disinfectant and iodine to produce a sense of normalcy.

Pancake Sunday was the brainchild of an American shrink who conducted his ministry in silence, only ever showing up to mix

---

* "Green on blue" refers to an attack made on one's own side by forces regarded as neutral.

and fry and wash up but never to speak. No one seemed to know quite who he was, except that his name was Eugene and that he recently qualified, and that he earned his keep courtesy of the Freud squad.* If his vow of silence was intended as an inducement to get others to talk, it was working, except that they didn't talk to him. This didn't seem to bother Eugene as he fixated on his gizmos—a hot pad and stick of butter, frying pan, whisk and bowl, spatula and pilfered carton of long-life milk—the docs his grateful flock.

Bomber and Hawkeye were first to bat. They sat down to a paper plate stacked three-high with buttermilk pancakes, a half inch of butter stick and maple syrup and hash browns and scrambled egg fished out of the Styrofoam container in which they had been smuggled out of Fort Leatherneck at sunrise.

Meanwhile, on the intensive care unit, a teenage triple amputee had lost the will to live. Without the use of his two legs, one of his arms, his right eye, and the best part of his scrotum, he had little to look forward to. His only window to the soul hadn't the slightest trace of resolve or hope. As Dante would put it, he wasn't dead, and yet nothing of life remained. His older brother had been transferred to Kandahar's neurosurgery unit with major head trauma. Both were playing outside when they stumbled on an explosive, making for an increasingly familiar story: whether homemade or Soviet spawned, bombs cannot tell friend from foe, child from adult, Tom from Dick from Harry. The boy hadn't had a single visitor since his arrival a week ago and was fated to take in life on the ward through his one remaining eye.

"It sounds harsh," Hawkeye said, "but the kind thing would be to put a pillow over his head and shoot the poor sod."

---

* Medical slang for psychiatrists.

Things didn't look all that much brighter for a little girl in the adjacent bed. Her beautiful black curls had been shorn off to treat multiple frag wounds to her zippered head and face. She'd had precisely one visitor in five days, though it is unclear whether he came specifically for her or simply stopped by while calling in on someone else.

Four beds down a blond, bushy-haired US soldier sat propped up against his pillows, shot through his left calf during yesterday's patrol. It was a clean flesh wound, washed out with the use of sterile cotton swabs and water. The procedure seemed simple enough and not unlike cleaning out a bit of pipe: one shoved the rag in one end to retrieve it from the other, and pulled it from side to side several times before running water through the cavity and filling it up with a clean bit of cotton for closing the next day. He refused to be stretchered in on arrival, and limped from the ambulance to resus instead, his face and hair covered in fine desert dust. He'd be back with his unit within a couple of days. For the moment he seemed content to peruse *FMH*'s 100 Sexiest Women of 2010, pilfered from the Doctors' Room, and frit away the hours.

THE EARLY MORNING delivery the next day involved a peculiar trio: a local contractor with the blade of a circular saw stuck in the bone midway through his right forearm, a man of unknown origin with gunshot wounds to his chest and head, and an Afghan with a crushed foot nowhere thicker than a fifth of an inch and double the width as a result. The last attracted a fair bit of interest. Everyone wanted to know: how in the heck did he get a foot that fucking flat? The victim, when asked, was evasive, but suspicions were that it had been run over by something heavy, perhaps a tank, flaring out as it did like a witch broom. The thing would have to come off but not before the crew had been rallied around for a look-see.

A similar prospect was facing our contractor. Nearly every major vessel in his right forearm had been severed, and without the benefit of a vascular specialist, it was unlikely to survive. His travel companion with the head and chest wounds was sent in for a CT scan, where it quickly emerged that the hole in his head had no matching exit wound. He wasn't to regain consciousness and let off comfortably with the use of opiates.

"Had he been a British soldier, we might have kept him alive until his family would have had a chance to say their goodbyes," Bomber had said, "though the upshot would have been the same either way."

The atmosphere in theater was glum. Hawkeye wandered in to check on the saw-blade victim being prepped for surgery. A scan showed the cut to be too deep and dirty for the arm to be salvaged, and so it was to be flung onto the burn pit together with the flat foot. The latter's proprietor meanwhile was well into his procedure, the skin flaps on his shin ready to be folded back over the remaining stump and sewn together. Fernsby and Jerrycan were scrubbing up for the arm amputation. Hawkeye, having little else to do, struck up a conversation with one of the scrubs.

"All right?"

"Same shit, different day."

"Need anything?"

"Reason to live," she said, not looking up, and not trying to be funny. Suzy was a fixture of the theater team and as such put in longer hours than anyone else. For even when the surgeons have done their bits there's still the cleaning up: yellow-bagging whatever goes into the incinerator, with everything else going into white sacks; disinfecting tables and floors with chlorinated water; ensuring surgical tools are collected and sterilized; stocking up on used items; and making sure the right surgical kit is at the ready for the next operation. She coated the offending arm in iodine as part of the surgical prep.

"A reason to live," Hawkeye replied. "Now wouldn't that be something?"

Brigadier General Malham Wakin wrote, "It is because we view life to be so precious that we can so readily agree that the profession whose principal function is to preserve life deserves our approbation." It's not entirely surprising then that many medical professionals experience their profession as a "calling" in much the same way clergy do: their ambitions serve a purpose other than careerism. The medical profession channels this higher calling into several values and principles that medical professionals are expected to uphold. The prioritization of patient care is embedded in the Hippocratic oath, and many medical schools today still hold ceremonies where graduates swear an updated version of it. In the UK, these updated versions are usually directly linked to the core values and principles for the medical profession set out by the General Medical Council in its *Good Medical Practice* guide. Among other things, "making the care of your patients your first concern," "providing a good standard of practice and care," and "complying with systems to protect patients" are key principles that medical professionals expect to enact.

Implied here is a professional culture that takes systems, protocols, and techniques very seriously. This was particularly evident in pre-deployment training for surgeons and anesthetists, which was predominantly technical in nature. This general technical focus is designed in part to desensitize doctors to emotions that may interfere with their ability to provide the best possible patient care. In medical training, emotions have long been considered potential impairments to decision making and the effective exercising of one's duty. Thus, through their technical training, the medical profession's higher purpose of acting in the interest of patient care becomes embodied in their technical ability to heal people. This provides practitioners with a clear sense of purpose and agency that is singularly focused on the patient and embodied in systems, protocols, and techniques.

This professional context socializes medical professionals into understanding their work identities as those who pursue a higher, noble purpose; who are there "to make a difference"; who achieve technical mastery through hard work and protocol; and who can maintain composed detachment at all times. This context may help explain how the doctors and nurses in Camp Bastion viewed themselves and their work, amplifying the dissonance between what they expected and desired as normal practice on the one hand, and, on the other, what they actually experienced on the ground in relation to an organizational context that, at least occasionally, appeared to force them to compromise on patient care and a cultural context that seemed blind to the inhumanity they encountered.[5] As so often in war, they found themselves at the receiving end of the effects of conflicting narratives—fabricated and perpetuated by politicians and the Taliban, institutions medical and military, Afghan civilians and folks back home—yet without a story line of their own to help them make sense of *their* experience.

5

Legs

B rook and I were chewing the rag in opposing beds in our two-by-five-meter, undecorated Tier Two room. We'd been room-mates for a couple of weeks, and Brook's time was nearly up. Two identical faux cherrywood wardrobes faced each other just off center. Aside from the odd wire hanger and spare blanket, they stood abandoned. A small bedside table with drawers provided a resting place for books we packed but would never read, a water bottle, alarm clock, spare change, and other tidbits. The drawers held the residue of residents past: a soiled sex mag, rubber band, paper clips, ballpoint pen, and a box of pills labeled "Man Up Tablets" to be taken "three times daily when necessary for manning up." Inside it were white tablets—vitamin tablets, most likely. I pocketed the box. Other than that, the room was soulless. Brook's duffel sat at the foot of his bed, mine on an unoccupied third bed, our worldly belongings a pitiful lot.

Brook was in a melancholy mood tonight and, privately, very critical of the efforts expended in Iraq and Afghanistan. Though he had been born in a military family, or because of it, he struggled to make sense of the war.

"We shoot them and then say here you go, here's a plaster, and then leave them to it. No matter who shot whom and why or who set off the explosives, when you get injured as a local you're done for." The Afghans, he told me, are held to local standards—after all, this is their country and their infrastructure—and any treatment beyond emergency surgery is referred to local hospitals in Lashkar Gah or Kandahar. He despaired of having to feed injured Afghans daily into a second-rate health care system where levels of care were several standard deviations removed from Bastion's, thinking it little wonder their chances of recovery were compromised as a result.

His wife and kids would never understand what he'd been through over the past five weeks, and other than people here, he wouldn't know whom to talk to. He spoke of the fear faced by soldiers before going on patrol, saying some throw up before they have to go out, or pump themselves up with push-ups before strapping on their gear and heading for the base's exit and the flatlands beyond, with the bugs and the bombs.

"Did you go to the repatriation ceremony?" he asked me.

"Yup. You?"

"No. It's hard enough seeing them in theater let alone stand there to be told all about who they were and what they meant to their regiment."

"..."

"You don't believe, do you?"

"Not really."

"Agnostic?"

"Sort of."

"..."

"It's complicated."

"MINE STRIKE." The MERT doctor called out to those gathered in resus, a tad out of breath for having legged it from the ambulance to beat the gurney.

"Injuries are: left below-knee amputation, frags to the right knee, frags to the right arm, lower arm all covered by a first field dressing, significant frags to the face. Upper lip's completely gone. He thinks his nose has gone as well. He's been maintaining his airway throughout. Observations on the cap have been: speaking, sats have been 100, tachycardic* 120 to 140, a good radial pulse† throughout; treatment-wise pre-hospital he's had 50 mg of ketamine, he's also had IM morphine and a benzyl pen. His name is Jack."

The gurney was wheeled in and placed next to the bed in Bay 1. Hawkeye was the attending surgeon in charge of the primary survey.

"Hi, Jack," Hawkeye said. "Nice to have you here and comfy. You just stay where you are. What we're going to do now, all right, is to move you onto your side, your right side, put something under your back, and then slide you onto another table, all right? So you just hang in there. You'll just feel us moving you and don't have to do a thing." The emergency care team would take their cues from Hawkeye for the next ten minutes or so.

"At the moment we're just untying you because you're strapped to a stretcher," Hawkeye told Jack. "Any second now you'll be lifted onto your right-hand side and just gently rolled."

The logroll caused Jack to whimper.

"Well done. Good lad."

"Stick your tongue out for me, will you?" the anesthetist said.

"Have I got a tongue?" Jack asked. His voice was distorted for the bloody bandages around his head and face.

"You've got a tongue."

---

* When the heart rate exceeds the normal resting rate.
† The heartbeat as felt through the walls of the radial artery at the wrist.

"Is it all there?"

"Your tongue is all there, yes. You'll be all right for the ladies."

"Jack, take a nice deep breath for me, will you? Good man," said Hawkeye. "Good expansion both sides. I need four more deep breaths of you so I can listen to your chest. Good man. Good air entry, all four quadrants, both sides."

Hawkeye continued: "Jack, apart from your face, does anything else hurt?"

"My left leg."

"Your left leg, okay."

Turning now to his colleagues, Hawkeye said: "There is a first field dressing on his right arm covering the hand and forearm. He's got a penetrating wound on the inside of his right upper arm. He's got a penetrating wound on the ulnar border of his right forearm."

"Jack, we're just cutting your trousers off, okay, or what's left of them. Is there any pain in your belly?"

"No."

"Good man. Jack, you're just going to feel me touching your tummy all right. Any serious illnesses or operations in the past?"

"Yeah . . . a suicide bomber two years ago."

"A what, sorry?"

"Got blown up two years ago."

"Okay."

" . . . "

"Are you allergic to anything?"

"No."

"Any tablets or medicines?"

"No."

Hawkeye told the staff: "He's got some fragment wounds around his left knee. He's got some bruising and some superficial lacerations on his scrotum."

As Jack began to moan, Hawkeye asked him whether his arm was sore.

"We know you've taken a bit of a twatting on your head and your left foot, and so that we can have a good look at you and sort you out, the plan is to pop you off to sleep and then nothing will hurt. We'll do whatever is required to make you better. You're doing really really well."

Jack moaned as the anesthetist changed his mask.

"So you ended up in the shit a few years back, did you?"

"Was doing this two years ago," Jack replied. "Got blown up by a fucking suicide bomber.

"..."

"For fuck's sake, what the fuck am I doing this shit for?"

"..."

"Can't even have a fucking tab,* can I, cause I've not got a top lip . . . for fuck's sake."

"I tell you what, someone will get you a tab when you're all sorted."

"The way I feel about my face I might as well stick it up my arse."

"You'll be fine, big man."

"Take those nice deep breaths, Jack," the anesthetist piped in as he prepared to insert a breathing tube.

"..."

"Intubated. Good air entry. Both sides."

And with that, Jack was wheeled to CT for a scan of his face and head. Hawkeye and the team peeled off, some for coffee, others to scrub. By the time Jack woke up, he'd be at Queen Elizabeth Hospital in Birmingham, surrounded by family and friends.

---

* Slang for cigarette.

IT'S THE KIDS that depress. Doctors tell me they're the toughest to treat, even as they rarely cry and are beautiful to behold with fine features and sun-kissed complexions not yet sucked dry by decades of conflict. Their hair varies in color from black to light brown, as do their irises, occasionally set in big round eyes with strong elongated eyelashes. Are these kids any less scared than their elders going into surgery? Their injuries are no less severe and, one would assume, no less painful. Then why is it they don't howl like grown men do?

The first casualty of the day was a local police officer with a hole through his right foot. Suspicions were that it was self-inflicted, its being far too cleanly placed for a plausible alternative. Presumably the man could not believe his luck when he was plucked from one or other inferno and dropped by helicopter onto a clean set of linens. No sooner had he been placed on the operating table, however, than a 270-pound former Estonian judo champion-cum-anesthetist jabbed an inch of hypodermic needle straight into his callused heel and, as if to add insult to injury, decided to give him a general anesthetic in any case. This double-whammy had him knocked him out cold in minutes, well before his tears had a chance to dry.

More grisly was the arrival of a fubar* older than the first. His face had been stripped straight back to the skull with a fist-size hole where his nasal cavity should be. Apparently he had been spotted burying a homemade explosive when the damn thing misfired. He was laid out on an olive gurney, clearly conscious, flapping his arms upward and sideways as if trying but failing to prevent himself from drowning. Was this an insurgent keen to play his part in the war against the infidel? Was he a family man,

---

* Medical slang meaning "fucked up beyond all recognition."

forced to dig in a bomb at the threat of his loved ones getting hurt should he disobey? Or was he a farmer happening upon an explosive in his field? Did he selflessly cause the thing to blow up on him so as to prevent injury to our soldiers? As with so many questions generated by this terrible war, we would never know, and so long as we didn't know—fuck it—he would be a detainee.

Not for long, as it happened. At just after 1600 the old man took the answer to his grave. He might have set off on this journey much earlier had it not been for one of the US administrators requesting that his death please be postponed so as to give them time to complete the relevant paperwork. It seems things were easier administratively if he died a free man rather than the detainee he now was; and thus while his "release" was being processed through the usual channels, he lay in intensive care, killing time for the sake of managerial convenience.

The stories the docs tell each other are instructive. Hawkeye related the sad case of a girl during his last deployment to Afghanistan. As the youngest child it had been her job to light the kerosene lamps at dusk. This, he said, was common practice in Afghanistan, however unsafe or unimaginable this might be in the West. That night something went wrong and she got badly burned but survived. She arrived with 35 percent burns, maybe a bit more, he said, and was kept on the ward for far longer than usual. When she was well enough to be sent home, the hospital surrendered the girl to her parents, only to find out that when her fate was subsequently discussed at a family shura,* the view was that she was too

---

* Arabic for "consultation." The Quran encourages Muslims to decide their affairs in consultation with those who will be affected by that decision.

ugly to ever get married and too badly maimed to be able to work. And so, Hawkeye said, they starved her.

Southwark, in turn, told of a British nurse who had arrived in the hospital with severe burns. She had befriended a young boy, plying him with candies, until one day he threw a plastic bucket at her, dousing her in petrol and setting her alight. The Taliban, Southwark said, are not shy about using children to advance their interests, whether by forcing them to walk donkeys heavy with explosives toward the infidel or by leaving injured kids by the roadside as bait to attract a medevac helicopter.

I never did set out to investigate whether these stories were factually correct. To insist on doing so is to risk missing an altogether more relevant point: these are the tales related by medical staff to others, often those more junior, and it is these stories that play an important socializing function in bringing newcomers into the fold. And there are plenty of stories. When, upon my return to the UK, I shared my experiences with a senior, nonmedical, military officer, he volunteered his own. He talked of one particular day, when he was out with the troops patrolling a small village and they were asked if they could please help rescue a small girl stuck down a well. The family's only source of freshwater had caved in, and so they had decided that the girl, being the smallest, would be best placed to remove the debris. As she was let in the well and began the process of prying loose the rocks, however, the thing caved in further and the little girl got stuck. His troops tried but were not able to free her. And so, he said, she died upside down.

SMITTY, one of two operating room coordinators, was summoned to meet a visitor at reception. A US marine had called earlier to report the discovery of two partial legs belonging to Billy, one of the troops in his charge, and would it be all right if he dropped them off at the hospital? He and his troops had been told that if limbs could be reattached within six hours of an explosion, they'd have a chance of surviving. The legs had been cold too long, Smitty told him, and were probably too badly damaged to be reattached in any event, but the marine was not to be dissuaded and made his appearance soon after.

"I gather you've got something for me?" Smitty said, trying as best he could to avoid embarrassing his visitor by attracting the attention of others seated nearby. But the marine would have none of it.

"Billy's legs," he said and handed Smitty a floppy carton box that once upon a time held US army rations.

". . ."

"You be sure to fix him up, won't you?"

"Leave it with us."

"Billy's a quarterback, you know, when we get time to play. Has one hell of an arm."

"His arm's fine."

"You look after him now."

As soon as the marine took off, Smitty got hold of Ginger, a scrub nurse on his first-ever tour. They shared one of the eight-bed pods, and over the past three months Smitty had taken it upon himself to be Ginger's mentor and confidant.

". . ."

"What's this?"

"Legs. Used to belong to the guy in theater three."

"Well what the fuck am I supposed to do with them?"

"Walk them over to the incinerator, that's what."

". . ."

". . ."

"Sure whoever gave you this is gone?"

6

Apocalypse Now and Again

I don't suppose it is any coincidence that I was given a set of titles to read prior to deployment: *MASH* (Richard Hooker), *Catch-22* (Joseph Heller), *My War Gone By, I Miss It So* (Anthony Loyd), *The Bang Bang Club: Snapshots from a Hidden War* (Greg Marinovich and João Silva), *Unreasonable Behaviour* (Don McCullin), *Emergency Sex and Other Desperate Measures* (Kenneth Cain, Heidi Postlewait, and Andrew Thomson), *What It Is Like to Go to War* (Karl Marlantes), *On Killing* (Dave Grossman), *Meditations in Green* (Stephen Wright), and *Heart of Darkness* (Joseph Conrad). I was instructed to consume them. They'd been particularly successful at portraying the lived experience of war, I was told, even if not from a medic's perspective, and I remember wondering whether this was really what the experience of the docs would be like, what they wish it were like, or what they'd like me to think it is like. Each book contains examples, and plenty of them, of the absurd, alongside the chaotic, sad, pointless, and outright strange. Michael Herr wrote of a colonel who had threatened to court-martial a spec 4 for refusing to cut the heart out of a dead Vietcong and feed it to a dog, and of a different colonel in the American Division who believed that every man under his command needed combat experience and so made the cooks take an M-16 each and go out on night patrol, and how one fated night all of his cooks got wiped out in a single ambush.[1]

Frank Ledwidge, until recently a UK military intelligence officer in Afghanistan, recalled the following in his own account of war:

> I had to interpret for one of the army handlers in a meeting with a Shi'a cleric, a mullah. The handler wanted to know what was said at Friday prayers—what the "atmospherics" were. "Ah," said the mullah, "there was a very holy atmosphere . . . it was as if the Imam Ali himself was there." Now, the Imam Ali is a seriously important figure for Shi'as, roughly comparable to St Peter or even Jesus. So when the handler asked in English: "Give me a full description of the Imam Ali," I did not translate it, but told the handler who the Imam Ali was. He was not sympathetic: "I ask the fucking questions; you translate." So I did. The mullah replied: "He died thirteen hundred years ago, so I don't know. Tell your friend I think he had a beard." I had many frankly embarrassing experiences like that, and they did us no good at all.[2]

Another of the recommended reads, and quite possibly the darkest of the lot, relates a similarly absurd incident, this time in Bosnia:

> The BiH [Bosnia and Herzegovina] had pioneered the first death-as-life weapon form south of Vitez late that autumn, filling the packs of two mules with explosives and rigging them to detonation cords before slapping them off towards the HVO [Croatian Defense Council] trenches. In true Bosnian style the animals, reluctant sehids [martyrs] began to graze in no-man's-land and after a while wandered back to the Muslim trenches. You did not even have to be there to get the grim joke.[3]

Then there is the absurdity of medical staff relying for their enjoyment on yet more gratuitous violence. Doctors, when not working, could often be seen watching Hollywood interpretations of modern warfare. *A Bridge Too Far, Apocalypse Now, The Deer Hunter, Platoon,* and *The Hurt Locker* were particularly popular, as were reruns of the American cult series *M.A.S.H.* The irony of watching fictionalized treatments of war in the midst of war's casualties seemed lost on, well, everyone.

EVERY NEW ARRIVAL would be announced by beepers suspended from drawstring surgical bottoms and passed around like cheap dates at the close of every shift. Those who concluded their shift handed the baton to those about to begin theirs in a ritual that invariably involved a gibe or two but rarely a smile. These bleepers would summon their bearers to resus, where the outside doors would be propped open in anticipation of gurneys, and before long be joined by others who would have picked up the heavy pulsating of the Chinook and, lost for anything else to do, threw their lot in with the rest. In doing so, of course, they risked turning resuscitations into clusterfucks, Hawkeye said, everyone turning up for every single trauma call.

All afternoon, eyes were fixed on a three-by-four-foot whiteboard, hung in the eight-yard subsection that divided resus and operating theater. On it, in dry marker, were the nationality, injury type, and priority level of incoming casualties, and opposite them the names of those responsible for their care: who would conduct the primary survey, who would be anesthetist, who would be in charge, who would do the blood and lab runs, and who would help do the logroll, draw blood, cut off combats, and take and read X-rays and ultrasound scans. Those casualties identified as Cat A were always the most serious, B and C less so, though all is relative. What registered as a Cat B in Bay Springs, Mississippi, or in Britain's Barnstaple might well slip out of the rankings altogether in Bastion.

One of the Cat A's that afternoon was Afghan. He arrived with a bloodied face and neck, and with injuries to his chest. Hawkeye was on the case straightaway. With the usual lack of detail on the circumstances of this find, and with the primary survey inconclusive, he called for order and told his team that in his view the guy should make a right turn (straight into the operating theater) for a rapid-sequence intubation. Given the extent of the damage to his face and chest, it was unclear whether a normal intubation would do the trick, and Hawkeye was keen to have sufficiently good lighting to perform an emergency tracheotomy if necessary. Meanwhile he would insert two chest-drains, one on each side, to empty the chest cavity of whatever free blood had accumulated inside it. As a rule of thumb, any liquid in excess of a liter and a half needed the chest to be opened up, said Hawkeye, so as to fix the bleeding inside out.

No one voiced objections, and the casualty was taken into theater, where Brook succeeded in his first attempt at intubating him. Hawkeye made two quick incisions, one on each side of the chest and below the armpit before pushing his index finger inside it past the muscles and ribs. As he pulled back, the expected trickle of blood followed, and he proceeded to insert the chest drains. Buoyed up by the ease of intubation, and keen to get their tuppence in, seventeen others soon joined Hawkeye and Brook around the operating table, turning the spectacle into a dog's breakfast.

Air Commodore Phil Soleski, in command of the hospital, had drifted in midway through his daily fitness routine, T-shirt and shorts moist with perspiration. It was he who made the ultimate call on matters of life and death or, as in the case of transfers to local hospitals, limbo.

Soleski had been summoned to make a call on how to proceed with Hawkeye's patient. The noisy carnival that greeted him did little to lift his prickly spirits, and his calls for quiet fell on deaf ears. It was left to Hawkeye to calm the torrent with a colorful scolding before outlining the plan: to take him to CT for a scan of his head, neck, and chest.

Noise seems to be an important cue in both resus and theater, presumably because it isn't always easy to see what is going on. Where injuries require the input of several orthopods, a couple of general surgeons, anesthetists, and supporting staff, noise levels act as useful indicators. If all goes well, noise should be at a minimum, and the whirring of the anesthetic machine distinguishable. Rising noise levels can be a bad sign: the patient may be misbehaving, or perhaps there are too many staff around the table to work effectively. The ensuing chaos was for Soleski to sort out.

While Hawkeye agonized about bleeding in the chest, the head injury proved worse than suspected. The question had become one of whether treatment would divert the course of nature and up the odds of survival, or whether he would be best left to ride it out on morphine. These life-or-death decisions were common in Bastion, yet required Soleski's blessing, and so he was called on once again to direct his flock of the capable but unhappy. The scans did nothing to help him make up his mind, and so he asked for the images to be wired to Kandahar for a second opinion by their neurosurgeon. Forty-five minutes on, Soleski having resumed his stint on the treadmill meanwhile, the neurosurgeon returned an amber-slash-red verdict, meaning chances of survival were slim. The Afghan was made comfortable and slipped effortlessly into the sweet hereafter.

Once nature had taken its usual course, his body was washed and bound in traditional fashion by two male nurses. The *gushl*, or traditional cleansing, is obligatory on all Muslims and repeated three times, or if necessary more often, so long as the tally adds up to an odd number. His nose and teeth were cleaned and hair combed. A cotton bandage, never silk for men, was wrapped around the head to keep the jaw shut, while another bound his ankles together. His arms were positioned next to the body, and all of it washed before being transferred to the morgue. Whereas Afghans are usually cleaned and wrapped up on the ward, behind screens, NATO troops are offered the solitude of air conditioning, and the companionship of those with strong enough stomachs to be able to wash, dress, and box up their fallen countrymen. The commitment of the lads managing the American morgue, adjacent to its British counterpart, is more impressive yet: they sleep with their dead as a matter of principle.

I looked on, wondering how it is that these Afghans continued to follow their God seeing all the shit they'd been through over the past few decades. Why would anyone wish to play any part in a proselytizing faith if it causes so much pain and injustice? Why submit to a religion that pits people against each other? Why would a benevolent, all-powerful and all-seeing God allow his creation to suffer and to inflict such terrible suffering? Is this the price of our so-called freedom to choose good or evil, a price paid not by those exercising their freedoms but by the very targets of their perversions, and where the only recompense is a childlike vision of an everlasting bliss where lion and sheep will lie together and pain will be no more? What the fuck is the lion going to eat?

I recalled G. K. Chesterton suggesting somewhere that for life to be worth living we need values worth dying for, a submission that seems to have been taken rather too earnestly here and may be part of the problem. I remembered the shallow comfort derived in youth from being told that any scorn suffered here and now surely paled in comparison to that suffered by our sweet Lord in his

time, and that one must not be put off but be steadfast even under
testing circumstances, and being given literature to read, and tent
meetings to go to, and sundown singsongs too, and prayers at Friday sundown, and slogans like "If God seems far away guess who
moved?" and "What would Jesus do?" and "If you die today where
will you be tomorrow?" and "Honk if you love Jesus" (yes and
screw you too); and Weeks of Prayer, and altar calls—oh God did
I feel queasy—burdened always with the obligation to proselytize,
to make disciples of all nations, baptizing them in the name of the
Father and of the Son and of the Holy Spirit, and teaching them to
obey, realizing all the while that "we stand on a mountain pass in
the midst of whirling snow and blinding mist, through which we
get glimpses now and then of paths which may be deceptive; if we
stand still we shall be frozen to death; if we take the wrong road
we shall be dashed to pieces"; we must be "strong and of good
courage" for "if death ends all, we cannot meet death better."[4]
If I have done away with God, as I keep telling myself, why then
do I keep fingering my fucking soul like an open fucking wound?[5]

"Ah pray for them is what Ah do." An American nurse, older
than the rest, had snuck up from fuck knows where. "Ah pray and
pray that God have mercy on their souls is the way Ah deal with
it, and Ah pray that our boys may be safe. Ah don't know much
theology and Ah don't pretend to understand but Ah do know that
God has His reasons and so Ah just pray that His will be done. We
can do no more now, can we?" Bothered by her sincerity, or the
intrusion, or because she reminded me of my own folk who blew
it in this department, I fucked off to join Ty in his newly cultivated
tomato patch outside, behind the Doctors' Room.

BACK IN THE OPERATING THEATER meanwhile yet another casualty
had arrived: a US marine with a gunshot wound to just above his

knee. What seemed trivial in comparison with the double amputee turned out to require major surgery since the bullet made merry with both vein and artery, necessitating grafting using existing vessels harvested from his healthy leg.

As the hour turned late and later still, the surgical team broke out in song, Ty first, the others hot on his heels. Surgeons and scrub nurses, ODPs and anesthetists, the theater coordinator, the guy from the blood bank, all joined in as Ty fronted a motley crew of off-pitch voices—

Is this the real life?
Is this just fantasy?
Caught in a landslide
No escape from reality

Shuffling past the choir of doctors in the long corridor were three suspected insurgents with minor injuries. They were brought to the ward blindfolded by a pair of strapping US marines. Eat your heart out, Farrokh.*

JOCK TALKED of a rude awakening to the cruelty of war when, on his last tour of Afghanistan, he had been asked if he could help identify the perpetrators of a particularly callous attack on a school bus. Its cargo of children had been annihilated by gunfire. Not a single child survived, nor did the driver for that matter, leaving no witnesses. Question was, did the bullets belong to coalition forces or to the insurgency? Since Bastion did not have a pathologist, Jock had been asked to do the unpalatable by recovering the

---

* Freddie Mercury was born Farrokh Bulsara in the Sultanate of Zanzibar.

bullets so they could be sent off for forensic analysis. He described unclasping the metal door to a shipping container, the air inside uncirculated, stale, hot. And there they were, in a bundle. There was little to indicate which limb belonged to which torso, and so Jock had to bend over one child to try to pry out the slugs from the one under it, and others underneath that one. It is a memory that, he said, makes him wake up still in cold sweat.

> *It had the earth black with congealed blood and littered with abandoned guns, packs, and tunics; everywhere severed body parts, splintered bone fragments, cartridge boxes; riderless horses nosing about among the corpses; faces twisted in the convulsions of death; wounded men crawling toward pools of bloody mud to slake their thirst; and avid Lombard peasants scurrying from corpse to corpse, to rip the boots from the feet of the dead. . . . Dressed in his increasingly bloodstained white linen suit, he wandered among the dead and dying, crammed into the nave of the village church, passing out cigars in the belief that the whiff of a good Havana would allay the stench of putrefying wounds.* [6]

ANOTHER GUNSHOT WOUND turned up not long after the American had been dispatched to intensive care. He was a member of the Afghan National Police and had yet another conveniently placed hole in his foot. His story, the interpreter told us, is that someone shot him from ten meters away.

"Looks more like he shot himself," the radiologist said, as he scrutinized yet another perfectly placed wound right in the fleshy bit between the toes. Traces of gunpowder residue on his leg suggested that the man might well have made a choice between this and joining the Taliban, and took matters into his own hands.

Self-harm isn't the sole preserve of Afghans, however. More troops have been evacuated from non-battle-related injuries (of the six thousand–plus men and women who were evacuated between 2001 and 2012, just over two thousand were "wounded in action") than from combat wounds, and while only a small proportion of those injuries are likely to have been self-inflicted, estimates run as high as 10 to 15 percent. A slug to the foot is the method of choice for locals. NATO troops, when pushed, seem more likely to opt for self-inflicted cuts, broken limbs, or poisoning. The chief cause need not be cowardice, of course. Much of the self-harm seems to relate to support troops, rather than those on the front line, and triggered by relationship problems, including those back home. Is it because they have more time to sit and fret than those on daily patrols? Or is it a reluctance to put their lives at risk for a war that is scheduled to end soon anyway, and so why throw good after bad?[7]

ANOTHER EARLY MORNING patrol and another set of victims. First to bat was a casualty who never so much as made it into the Chinook alive, even as the MERT team began a course of CPR straightaway and was at it still when scurrying him into resus. But it wasn't to be. One of the contributing causes declared itself pretty promptly once the American had been logrolled onto the table: not one of the four tourniquets attached to his stumps had been fastened tight enough to stem the outflow of blood. In the pandemonium following the explosion, his buddies hadn't remembered to double-check that they were on tight and so left him to bleed out even as they rushed him to the helicopter; a double pity, as soldiers are often told that so long as they make it to the MERT they will live, and the heavy slugging of the Chinook's twin rotors thus comes as an immense relief, or should, in any case.

"Bloody Americans," griped one of the MERT docs. "Can't even apply a simple tourniquet."

But Hawkeye would have none of it.

"You try being out there when the shit hits the fan and you're being shot at and having to run through a minefield trying to protect your mate and yourself and carrying fifty kg's on your back and having to carry another hundred and ten kg's on a gurney for two fucking miles to where the MERT has landed and then being told that you didn't fasten the fucking tourniquets tight enough so your mate's dead. Just imagine what that will do to you. That will fucking do your head right in!"

A second DOA wasn't far behind. Surgeons watched from behind the yellow line as the curtains were drawn around.

"Would have been a fantastic case," Southwark said to Weegee, "and now you've ruined it."

"But the guy is dead," Weegee replied.

"Doesn't matter. There's a bone to be fixed, so let me fix it."

Smitty was much less sanguine looking on. With the operating theaters in his charge, it was his responsibility to make sure all the surgical preps were in place prior to each operation and that tables were allocated efficiently, and he is vastly more capable than his rank would suggest.

"I always make a point of looking at each injury that comes in," he told me as he readied a second theater. "No matter how miserable or unpleasant, I want to be shocked by the stuff that comes in, just to remember that this is not normal, that there is a different world out there."

A glum band of brothers, the docs trundled back to their lair to feast on *Apocalypse Now*, a Coppola masterpiece loosely based on Conrad's *Heart of Darkness*. Its protagonist is guilty of unspeakable crimes. A telling, and rather infamous, scene shows a swarm of American helicopters advancing like locusts on a Vietnamese settlement to the brass tones of Wagner's "Ride of the Valkyries." It didn't seem to strike any of those glued to the telly as ironic that less than a klick away their own Apaches were taking off on similar missions, armed to the teeth with AGM-114 air-to-surface Hell-fire missiles and with a much-feared canon between their landing gear. It would quite literally have taken no more than stepping outside of the Doctors' Room and onto the wooden patio to fast-forward forty years to a similar scene. Alas, the patio door was closed shut, and the telly on, and they around it in a half circle, "near beer" and homemade cookies and ginger cake and chocolate to hand.

"My favorite line's coming up," Southwark said excitedly. "Wait for it ... ah, 'I love the smell of napalm in the morning.' Absolutely first class that is."

Four bleepers let rip in unison: a Cat A was on its way, and would all please make their way to resus without delay. Taking their cue from the white dry marker board, the team rallied around, those not selected loitering in the vicinity disappointed, and behind the yellow line. This painted line, about an inch or so wide, was designed to separate the team tasked with treating a patient from those with little else to do. With the casualty still in transit, the whiteboard had already identified him as American and a double amputee.

His legs were badly buckled thanks to yet another homespun combination of fertilizer sourced from neighboring Pakistan, a set of AAA batteries, fuse, and detonator, a few feet of wiring, shrapnel, and a pressure plate. Lying as he did on the white-and-green-papered faux-leather bed, he was blissfully unaware of Ty sawing through his left femur with Southwark prepping the other leg. His right tibia fibula combo had come off during the log-roll in resus, leaving one of the nurses holding rather more than she'd signed up for.

The other leg looked perfectly healthy except for a gaping hole where his knee should have been. In an increasingly familiar limbs-in-bins routine, the unsuspecting lower leg was dropped in a yellow bucket and stuck out foot first like a periscope. The ortho-pods rid the remaining stump of its dead, or dying, flesh. It is the stuff that looks like uncooked hamburger that wants removing, Hawkeye had said.

The next double amputee was more distressing for being a small child. The explosive had torn deeply into his buttocks and shat-tered his pelvis. A large incision from just below the boy's ster-num and around his belly button down to his pubis made for a big enough hole for Bomber to have a good look around. The damage was extensive, he said. As he handled the various organs, examin-ing each in turn, he said it was kind of difficult to distinguish what was salvageable from the stuff that wasn't.

Soleski meanwhile had dragged his sweaty self back in from yet another fitness regime, took a good look, and voiced his opinion that this type of injury was not survivable in Afghanistan, and did anyone have any objections, he wondered.

"If so, say so, or else forever hold your peace." He faced the gas-sers, slashers, and scrub team. Everyone knew full well how this would play out.

"Right, so how about making the kid comfortable and giving him some dignity," he had said before the crowd thinned out and the sky-blue privacy curtains were wheeled in from the ward. As for the little boy, that was by the by. He would never know what hit him.

> *When you're wounded and left on Afghanistan's plains,*
> *And the women come out to cut up what remains,*
> *Jest roll to your rifle and blow out your brains*
> *An' go to your Gawd like a soldier.*[8]

My head spinning, I sat down behind the communal desktop in the Doctors' Room to pen my wife a long-overdue e-mail, followed by one to Bud:

From: Rond Dr M. E. J. de
To: Rond R. M. de
Subject:

Dear Roxana:

Today was a bad day: 18 casualties of which two died (some people here call them Angels, when they do saying things like "we had two angels today"), 7 had amputations and 5 had major debridements. One was a 7-year-old girl with major soft tissue injuring to her legs and arm (and even face). The Americans have been particularly hard-hit recently, and it is terrible to see how destructive IEDs really are. Guys come in daily with one or two limbs blown off, which can lead to high amputations, sometimes an amputation to an arm to top it all off. The docs debride the dead tissue, pack them up and ship them home. Many of the casualties are Afghan. They include children. Tonight they took a 12-year-old boy back into the operating room because he would have otherwise bled to death. He already had both legs amputated, and a badly damaged arm, had a laparotomy done, and an eye taken out. He is infectious and is not expected to make it.

I don't know why I really am here. I hope there'll be some merit to it all. Right now I'm not sure. I also feel further from God than ever, finding it difficult to pray.

From: Rond Dr M. E. J. de
To: Bud Popsugar
Subject: This will amuse you

Just had the most God-awful day with shite-loads of misery flocking in only to find in my inbox a long spiel by a senior colleague back home about the importance of placing our work in "top-tier jour-nals," and listing them as if we didn't know, and how we weren't here to solve all the world's problems but to get our research rating up. . . . God almighty, how much further can one get from the dark reality of life?

7

Boredom

The last four days had been unusually quiet, which bred an ugly mood of impatience and agitation. To help lift the spirits, tonight had been designated "poker night." Ty was making the most of the slow day by teaching Doo Rag how to play Texas hold 'em, using cards and props from an old, beat-up, duct-taped cookie tin.

"Sure you never played this, huh?" Ty had asked, a plug of tobacco tucked underneath his lower lip.

"How 'bout a game for real money tonight?" Practice was grinding. Doo Rag, despite his book smarts, took a while to get with the program. Ty spat into an empty Coke can every so often as he navigated his fellow American through the intricacies of poker. Doo Rag's beginner's mistakes would have left Ty hopeful of a lucrative evening.

"Doing great, buddy."

"Three of the same is a full house?"

"Only if the other two match, otherwise it's three of a kind."

"What if three of the cards are in sequence, just not the same suit?"

"Then that's nothing. But if you can make up two pairs and I can too we may have to use a kicker."

"A what, sorry . . . ?"

Boredom hung in the air like a peasouper that wouldn't lift except for the briefest of periods. In principle, this should have been good news—after all, no one was getting hurt—except that it left the docs with nothing meaningful to do. There was the occasional bit of exercise in a muggy gym to provide a temporary lift, or reading or daytime television, but little to take pride in, to feel productive about. And so they found themselves pining for work to come in, even if this invariably came at the expense of someone else getting hurt.

But boredom extracts its pound of flesh in other ways too. Left with little or nothing to do, Hawkeye, Southwark, Fernsby, Buster, Ty, Bomber, Oskar, and Doo Rag have begun to criticize each other's handling of patients and treatment and discharge decisions.[1] Hawkeye accused Oskar of removing a perfectly healthy appendix. Bomber faulted Doo Rag for opting against a tracheotomy where he was sure one was warranted, even if Doo Rag was proved correct the next morning.

"Better lucky than sorry," Bomber had responded dismissively. Everyone was ganging up on Hawkeye for neglecting a scan after an emergency procedure and as a result missing serious injuries to a casualty's back. Left to their own devices these docs become broody and aware of the relative futility of some of what they do here, particularly when it comes to providing emergency treatment for Afghans whose chances of recovery were badly compromised as soon as they were transferred to local hospitals, or so they think.

"Says he's bored, says he'd rather run around the woods ducking gook bullets than sit on his hemorrhoids reading Batman comic books."
"Kline is not well."
"Major Brand laughed in his face, said the unit was under strength and every swinging dick was needed just in case quote the balloon

should go up unquote. So Kline stands there wheezing, says, 'Well sir,
then with your permission I guess I'll just go back to my room and
jack off.'"

"*Funny little Kline.*"

"*I don't know. He wants to play soldier, they should let him. What*
should we care? We got lieutenants falling out our crack."[2]

Poker made for a welcome diversion from BBC sports coverage. In preparation for poker night, the mock games were moved
into an empty operating theater with surgical stools drawn
around, the bed doubling as poker table. Southwark, Fernsby,
and Jerrycan joined the gang. Ty sat at the head. Convinced that
there was a killing to be made, he did not realize that Doo Rag
had been coming along a hell of a lot more quickly than he let
on, so much so in fact that Ty was busted at the end of a long
night of playing.

Croft, Staff Sergeant Croft, was feeling another kind of excitement
after the next row of cards was turned up. He had been drifting sul-
lenly until then, but on the draw he picked up a seven, which gave him
two pair. At that instant, he had a sudden and powerful conviction
that he was going to win the pot. . . .

"*Bet two pounds," Croft said.*

Wilson threw two into the pot, and then Gallagher jumped him.
"*Raise you two." That made it certain Gallagher had his flush, Croft*
decided.

He dropped four pounds neatly on the blanket. "And raise you two."
There was a pleasurable edge of tension in his mouth. . . .

. . . Croft, containing his excitement, looked about the half-dark
hold, gazed at the web of bunks that rose all about them, tier on tier.
He watched a soldier turn over in his sleep. Then he picked up his last
card. It was a five. He shuffled his cards slowly, bewildered, wholly
unable to believe that he could have been so wrong. Disgusted, he
threw down his hand without even checking to Wilson. . . .

"Ah'm makin' an awful mistake, but Ah'll see ya," Wilson said.
"What ya got, boy?"[3]

PERIODS OF GREAT intensity followed periods of boredom in which it
was nevertheless impossible to relax. After a morning of e-mails,
expressions of unhappiness, banter, and armchair sports, courtesy of the BBC, resus kicked into gear at 1628. Five casualties had
arrived: a US marine with a gunshot wound to his forearm; an
Afghan with a bullet hole through to the ear; a UK rifleman with
kidney stones; an Afghan insurgent with bullets in his shoulder,
arm, and thigh; and a local contractor with a gunshot wound
to the chest, quickly reclassified as a "person of interest," meaning that, like any insurgent, he would be assigned his very own
chaperone twenty-four seven, unable to poop without a uniform
looking on.

Hawkeye and his Estonian colleague, Oskar, were tasked with
the multiple GSW. Oskar took the lead only to discover that what
looked like bullet holes were really ball bearings shot clear through
the torso, arms, and legs. Homemade explosives were becoming
difficult to detect and, as seemed to have been the case here, could
be activated remotely, pulverizing whatever animal, vegetable, or
mineral happened to be in the kill zone at the time.

Things took a turn for the worse when Oskar misread the man's
blood pressure for his pulse and decided on the spot that he was to
be taken into theater without further delay. This meant bypassing
CT or just the sort of thing that might have been useful in pinpoint-
ing where the diaspora of bearings had set up shop. The attending
anesthetist was aware, as he said with some misgiving afterward,
that the readings were likely to have been misunderstood but fig-
ured the screen was there for all to see, and when Oskar decided
on an emergency laparotomy, he thought fuck it. As the surgeons

peeled off to scrub, he was still seething at Oskar's knee-jerk decision but choosing to self-censor nonetheless, telling me later that he just didn't feel up to a confrontation with someone whose English was so fucking poor, and so drank the Kool Aid instead.

Had he not worked himself into the operating room and stuck with what he was supposed to be here for, he would have already hanged himself, he said. The critical-care air support team had not provided him with enough to do to feel good about, and so he ended up muscling his way into one of the operating theaters when and where he could. He said he'd rather do anything other than what he'd been tasked to do, so long as it kept him busy. With only nine short flights a week, on average, to ferry patients to local clinics, there just wasn't enough work for him and his nursing staff. Little work might be good in principle, but the mind-numbing boredom it induced was destabilizing and bred resentment like mold in a petri dish. His nurses certainly did look the part as they sat around limply in a mostly empty C-CAST* office, except for a couple of boxes, a kettle and tea-making paraphernalia, and the odd bit of chick-lit. And even with the muscling in, he still had too much free time to know what to do with. With too much downtime people get mischievous, he said.

The laparotomy meanwhile had uncovered a badly perforated bowel and stomach and bits of metal lodged in the liver, all of which took a good while to sort out. With the belly packed, Hawkeye found another four holes in the man's back, a couple in his hip and left arm, and an angry-looking right arm with yet more holes. A scan would have easily picked up these injuries, and a couple of orthopedic surgeons might have been drafted in to work on the

---

* Controller Communication and Situation Awareness Terminal.

limbs while Oskar and Hawkeye were elbow-deep into the belly. As is, the procedure tied up the theater's resources for far longer than necessary.

Sloppy Joe did the rounds taking pizza orders for the usual "Friday night pizza night" at a tenner a pop. While not everyone partook every Friday, most did, sending Joe off to procure a stack of pizzas from the makeshift Pizza Hut–KFC combo. Everyone else repaired to the Doctors' Room, where *Wedding Crashers* provided the ideal background to Hawkeye's wounded pride. Oskar, as usual, had meandered off back to his sauna but not before a young nurse had popped her head around the door to say that an Afghan had admitted himself with three months' worth of persistent pain in his bowels and unable to get an erection. Would Hawkeye mind taking a look? But Hawkeye wasn't interested. An Afghan who can't get it up wasn't high on his list of priorities.

We headed out to the KFC–Pizza Hut combo for a cold drink.

"The lads on my ship used to cheat on their girlfriends and then show up to my surgery for me to check their bits and give them the all clear," Hawkeye said. "And sometimes they want the meds even if nothing is wrong with them, as if the meds take away the guilt, and I had to tell them that no amount of antibiotic will ever fix that. And then when it came to our stopover in Thailand, the lads could get a blow job or shag for twenty bucks or a fiver if they didn't mind the sheets not being changed, or they'd get together and rent a few girls for a week at a time and hole up in an apartment somewhere."

"   "
". . ."

"And then they'd wonder where all the STIs* come from."

---

* Sexually transmitted infections.

I SAT DOWN and wrote Bud an e-mail:

From: Rond Dr M. E. J. de
To: Bud Popsugar
Subject: Re:

Help me out here. A pretty nurse put a sticky note on my chest. "Cock," it says. What does that mean?

From: Bud Popsugar
To: Rond Dr M. E. J. de
Subject: Re: Re:

Well you know what Don Winslow would say. How sticky was the note?

From: Rond Dr M. E. J. de
To: Bud Popsugar
Subject: Re: Re:

Not sure how well versed Winslow is in the ways of the world beyond his imagination. I didn't know what to do so ended up leaving.

From: Bud Popsugar
To: Rond Dr M. E. J. de
Subject: Re: Re: Re:

It's certainly an unusual first move, I would say.

THE BOREDOM, when it hit, was wearisome. Everyone would rather it were busier, as I did too, but felt guilty for what that implied. Perhaps the force of their reaction to boredom—their unhappiness and their looking for work where none was available, their tendency to interfere with each other's work, or if not outright interfere then to become critical of it—is easier to appreciate when one bears in mind that there are few things more existentially disturbing than boredom. Kierkegaard thought it the root of all evil.

Heidegger likened it to a silent fog that drew people together into strange indifference.

The military is no stranger to boredom, not even on deployment to some of the most volatile, conflict-ridden regions in the world. Here is a journal entry from a US marine stationed in Afghanistan's Korengal Valley:

> We got bored a lot in between fighting. We dealt with it in our own ways. We played cards and we did anything to deal with the boredom. . . . We'd have five- or six-hour conversations about the technical difference between jam and jelly. But times you always had a feeling in the back of your throat, something like, "It's a little eerie. Why is it like this? This is war. It's not supposed to be like this. Nobody is bothering us, we're just taking it easy. Tanning." Sometimes you want to fight so bad, just to pass the time. I mean you could get into a fight, fighting for five or seven hours, and it's just a blink of an eye. But you could be playing poker for twenty minutes, and it takes forever. So, yeah, people would start wishing fights.[4]

Bored to tears, they resorted to killing a cow:

> Sergeant Al and Hoyt had this crazy idea: "Hey, let's kill a fucking cow." There were cows walking through our shit, so Hoyt made a spear, and him and Lackley and a few other guys go up there and they pin this one cow in the corner and killed it. We didn't shoot it, because then we would have got caught—you just can't fire weapons off whenever we wanted—so Hoyt made a spear out of a tent pole and a Rambo knife. He taped the Rambo knife to the end of the pole, and gouged it, stabbed it a few times, and that was how the cow went down. We had rudimentary tools to decapitate this cow. We used a Christmas tree saw, so that got pretty gory, and then after we got the head off, everyone was so proud, and we're like, "All right, now how do we gut the thing?" None of us knew how to gut anything. I was like, "Yeah, now cut it down the middle. Watch the bladder!" After we gutted it completely, we used a lot of its meat,

and Lackley cooked up some steaks that were phenomenal. The Afghanis who owned the cow came up and said, "We know you killed our cow." Finally, Sergeant Patterson told him, "Listen, it got caught in the wire. We didn't kill your cow." They wanted money for it, and we're like, "We can give you some rice and beans and stuff that equal the same value of the cow, but we're not giving you money for the cow." They got all pissed off at us, but that was the best steak I ever had.[5]

In Camp Bastion's hospital, with idle time on their hands, the surgical staff became introspective. They seemed to feel callous for not caring more than they did. They worried about the futility of providing emergency treatment for locals only to hand them over to an inferior local health care system. Often, though rarely publicly, they questioned the point of this, or indeed any, war. As one of them wrote to me shortly after my return:

> Funny how there's so much and yet so little to be said. I have been in a number of conflict environments now: Ireland, gulf war 1991, Bosnia, Kosovo, Macedonia, Iraq, Afghanistan, Sierra Leone, Sri Lanka etc. Had the opportunity to revisit areas in Kosovo that had been cleaned up and rebuilt. Difficult to work out what all the fuss had been about.

With little or nothing else to preoccupy them, some doctors tried to create work for themselves or began to compete for new work, hoping others might be late or tied up in minor procedures, so they could bagsie the next major casualty. Sebastian Junger described the troops he embedded with as so bored on occasion that they prayed for enemy contact as farmers pray for rain.[6]

It was as if life was doomed to oscillate between busyness and boredom with little in between, where a sense of significance and futility could change rapidly and unpredictably and shift the balance between altruism and selfishness, pleasure and guilt, the thrill of warfare and cowardice. "In this kind of war," wrote Don McCullin, "you are on a schizophrenic trip. You cannot equate what is going on with anything else in life. . . . None of the real world judgments seem to apply. What's peace, what's war, what's dead, what's living, what's right, what's wrong? You don't know the answers."[7]

8

Christmas in Summer

A faux snowman sat parked in a wheelchair at the hospital
entrance, everyone geared up for a night of debauchery and
fancy dress and silly games and secret Santa on what the wards
had decided should be a midsummer Christmas. The absurdity of
Christmas in summer, of willy warmers and fluffy handcuffs, and
of an inflatable boner on a string bouncing softly with the wind,
all within a stone's throw of the dead or dying or wishing they were
dead, seemed wasted on the partygoers.

Today's early morning patrol passed without casualties. Given
that patrols take place at dawn and dusk when the sun is at its least
spiteful, this usually means all hands on deck twice daily. That is,
except for the odd Patrol Minimize* when excursions are halted,
either because of poor visibility or because something else takes
priority, as when all resources were directed, as they were the other
day, at rescuing a poor soldier who strayed from his base and was
found, and promptly dispatched, by insurgents.

---

* Means that troops on the ground should limit their exposure to the enemy
(often by confining themselves to their bases and avoiding the usual twice-daily
patrols).

"These ragheads must have thought Christmas came early," Hawkeye said. Patrol-free days give insurgents plenty of opportunity to dig in new explosives, meaning that the next few days can be particularly vicious as troops struggle to identify freshly upturned soil in an otherwise familiar, arid terrain not helped by the wind blowing topsoil all across it.

At around 1800, three Cat A's arrived by Chinook, all American. The first had accidentally set himself on fire when trying to burn a pile of rubbish dressed only in shorts and a T-shirt. By roster, and in the absence of blue canoes,* different soldiers are assigned the disagreeable task of incinerating bagged-up feces, some in advanced stages of putrefaction and perfectly flammable. Combats must be worn at such times, covering the arms and legs, meaning beach attire is a definite no-no. He came in covered in third-degree burns over 29 percent of his body, the bulk of it below the belt, and would be on a plane back home come midnight.

"Can you smell that?" Jock nudged me. "Damn, I love the smell of burned flesh."

As a plastic in a specialized burns unit back home, he had his treatment protocols pat down. These require the casualty to be wrapped in an antiseptic silver sulfadiazine dressing to help prevent infection, to which over half of burn victims would ordinarily succumb. The silver dressing has broad-spectrum antimicrobial properties to help prevent the onset of sepsis. The dressing, pricey though it is, also acts as an external seal such that the body's natural immunological responses are preserved, and is usually left on the burns for three days before redressing.

The soldier's two companions were victims of gunshot wounds, one serious enough to have required CPR treatment midair. He

---

* Military slang for portable toilets.

was wheeled into resus with an emergency doctor on his knees on top frantically pumping his heart, only for time to be called and his future decided nine short minutes later.

By the time Hawkeye and I arrived at the welfare tent, the Christmas party was pretty much done and dusted. A few stragglers lingered, shooting the breeze in Hawaiian shorts, tees, and Christmas hats, trying but failing to mimic the effects of intoxication. Hawkeye rested his eye on the merrymakers for a few moments, helped himself to one of a handful of lukewarm near beers, and buggered off into the night alone.

From: Bud Popsugar
To: Rond Dr M. E. J. de
Subject: Re: This will amuse you

Hi Mark,

Btw, I had to laugh when I read your correspondence with your colleague and wanting to bang your head against the table. Me too! Me too! Honestly, one of the hardest things is to keep a straight face and civil tongue when I hear otherwise perfectly sane adults take seriously something ordinary with all the attendant academic tools and then smile and accept applause as if they cured cancer. And of course I used to be one of them, which makes it even stranger. But here's the thing that may help you: Ethnography saved me from a life of academic dentistry. Writing about real people in real situations and constructing a narrative so others could appreciate/understand/empathize with "what it was like to" made all the difference in my career and in my life. Got me out of my head, out of the office, and into worlds that I otherwise wouldn't have known. You've already done that, too, and it can be your lifeline. Of course you will have to deal with insults from those who think writing stories is for children, but hey, who reads their screed anyway?

Your colleague may come around, but I doubt it. They are like Tea Party Republicans, in that most of them get to those jobs by being asshats and narcissists. At least mine was always nice about knifing you in the back. As my grand old Jewish mentor once put it: "Fuck 'em. And pass me the salt."

BROOK'S FAG SPRANG to life at 0514, the pulsating Chinook audible already against the higher-pitched purring of its trigger-happy chaperone. The combo was reassuringly familiar: a pretty lass and her fat friend, except that here the fat one is the more highly prized. The smaller AH-64 Apache is there to protect the MERT team but can struggle to keep up with the more powerful CH-47 Chinook. In a hurry, the twin-rotor helicopter can reach speeds of 196 mph. Originally designed back in the sixties, Chinooks have been deployed to transport troops and artillery and to facilitate medical evacuations, helped by their three large cargo hooks and wide loading ramp at the rear end of the fuselage. Boeing's other brainchild, the Apache, is smaller, nimbler, and features a distinctive nose with powerful sensors to provide night vision and help locate targets who, if unlucky, are given the once over by missiles and rocket pods located on its side wings.

Two American soldiers had been in contact with a roadside bomb, an accident that left one with a fractured pelvis and internal bleeding. The other had his legs torn off at the hip. Two Afghan casualties had frags to the face. Jock set out to harvest the fragments from the locals while Hawkeye prepared to open the belly of the amputee so as to stem the blood flow to the legs by tying off the vessels from the inside. Bomber and Doo Rag meanwhile had their hands full with the pelvic injury. Both Americans, if they hung on, would be flown home within the next few hours.

"WHY AM I NOT FEELING worse about all this shit?" Doo Rag said to no one in particular. He, Ty, and Fernsby were shooting the breeze in the Doctors' Room.

"About what?" Ty replied from behind his now familiar bulge.

"My dad was in Vietnam and he still sees stuff. I don't see fucking nothin'. So what does that make me?"

"I'm not sure anyone does here really," Ty said.

"It's a bigger deal for sure when it's one of our own," said Doo Rag.

"Kids can be tough, especially when they look like your own," Ty replied.

" . . . "

"These kids don't look anything like mine," said Fernsby.

"Some say the shit comes out afterwards," Doo Rag said. "That's what the decompression is for."

"You mean sitting down with a couple of cans of beer around a pool and no one you know to talk to when all you want is to be back home? Whose stupid idea was that then?" Hawkeye, wandering in, had caught the end of the conversation.

"I wouldn't worry about not feeling more badly. People react different to different circumstances. Ask anyone here and they'll tell you the same thing," Fernsby said. "To be honest, I feel far worse about having to put down my pooch just before the tour."

> *The thinking comes later, when they give you the time. See, it's not a base out in the desert, let us decompress a bit. I'm not sure what they meant by that. Decompress. We took it to mean jerk off a lot in the showers. Smoke a lot of cigarettes and play a lot of cards.*[1]

" . . . "

"What sort of dog was it?"

AN EIGHT-YEAR-OLD was misbehaving. She had been intubated inflight with the endotracheal tube pushed too far down her right lung, leaving her left lung without oxygen. Apparently it was an easy mistake to make, particularly when relying on a stethoscope midflight in a noisy Chinook. The right main-stem bronchus was an almost straight continuation, as opposed to the sharp left turn made by its twin, meaning that a tube pushed too far in almost always ended up inflating the right lung. Patients fared poorly because blood circulating to the left lung didn't pick up any oxygen as it resumed its journey through the body. The crew hadn't spotted their mistake and diagnosed her condition as a hemothorax. Blood had gathered between her lung and chest wall, or so they thought, and it was this that was preventing her left lung from properly inflating. They had been on the radio straightaway, suggesting Hawkeye prep a chest drain kit. No sooner did the girl come in, however, than cart and kit had vanished into thin air. After prepping another, Hawkeye made a small incision in the girl's chest and inserted his index finger in between her ribs but without the predicted liquid pouring out. An X-ray helped clear up the confusion, and the mistake was rectified by pulling the tube upward and into its proper place. The unused chest drain kit got trashed. Inserting a central venous line, meanwhile, had provided its own challenges. Three nurses had taken turns trying to get access, but prodding big-gauge needles into a tiny vessel had ruptured her subclavian vein, causing it to bleed into her chest.

"Whoever tried to push those big needles into those small veins should be shot," Bomber said, visibly angry.

When the issue arose in a subsequent morbidity and mortality meeting,[2] much was made of what went wrong and what should be done next time to make sure this wouldn't happen again. Weegee, who had coordinated the trauma call, said he hated these M&M sessions.[3]

"Everything looks straightforward with the benefit of hindsight, but it just isn't that easy in the moment. Truth is that everyone tries hard to do the right thing, especially when it involves a kid where everything is smaller, where the numbers look different, where everyone tries to do their best to save her. . . . All I want to tell them is: you weren't there, so get lost."

Wandering back to the Doctors' Room for a bit of respite, Hawk-eye and Southwark were met by an Afghan double amputee in a wheelchair rolling himself into the ward, followed on his heels by a companion who had the amputee's prosthetic legs flung over his shoulders like a couple of two-by-fours.

"Sometimes I try telling my family some of these things, but they don't understand," said Smitty, having joined me on my meandering. "Hell, *I* don't understand." He went on to tell me about a double amputee who had come in over Easter weekend. One of the legs had been attached by only a skin flap and came off during the usual logroll, just as had happened recently with a different casualty. The attending nurse, who'd been left standing with a leg in her arms, had asked one of Smitty's team to please take it away for disposal. As the lad made his way to the morgue, crossing the ambulance bay en route, he was met by Soleski and a nurse walking the other way, sporting bunny ears and carrying Easter eggs.

These surreal experiences can have a profoundly disorienting and dislocating effect on people because they temporarily expose our inability to give everything its rightful place.[4] Reality is as it seems, and therein perhaps lies the difficulty. It is the contrast between the human gravity of the situation on the one hand and the casual nature of everyday rituals and routines on the other that gives such experience a bizarre quality. We import rituals and routines to new settings from our lives back home precisely to create a sense of normalcy, even if these very imports often end up serving as stark reminders that life here is anything but normal. That not all is right. That so much of it is so wrong.

A BADLY BURNED baby had taken up three beds in intensive care for eight consecutive days with an infection so contagious that the beds on either side had to be kept free just to minimize the possibility of its spreading. Meanwhile a major military campaign was scheduled to kick off in forty-eight hours' time, and the hospital had been warned to expect up to sixteen new casualties per day. So what to do with the baby? The options facing Soleski and his team weren't brilliant: either he was left to die here or sent home to die there. He wouldn't be getting any better was the consensus. During the morning meeting, Jock offered to take the boy back to the operating room for another look. But his colleagues would have none of it: the baby was going home.

In an increasingly familiar routine, the white dry-marker board had six new arrivals on it, the nature and extent of their injuries and ETA a moving feast as the MERT worked their way through the injured in their Kevlar-and-metal flying tube. Three died en route, all Afghans. A fourth, a young American marine, was shot through the nose and so badly disfigured that he had been patched up and rerouted to the US for reconstructive surgery. Two others arrived with big bullet wounds to the chest. Hawkeye inserted a chest drain into the worst affected before ordering him into the operating room for a clamshell thoracotomy, or a rapid opening of the chest cavity by means of a long incision across the chest and below the nipples, cutting through the sternum so as to crack open the chest. It is a risky procedure, if only for the complexity of postoperative care. Infections are common, and breathing can become a painful pursuit for those on the receiving end.

Not long after this first lot was processed, another four Cat A's showed up on the doorstep, flown in from one of the forward operating bases where some emergency treatment was provided but not quite enough to do the job. Hawkeye's casualty, the whiteboard foretold, would come with a leg splint already attached. Upon arrival, however, no splint was to be seen.

"Is this your patient?" Hawkeye called out to the medic who wheeled him in and was about to make his escape.

"The guy I'm meant to have has a splint, and I certainly don't see anything like a splint on this one, how about you?" A flustered medic grabbed hold of the gurney and wheeled him into the next bay, and all casualties were re-dispensed in a game of musical chairs.

Two of the four casualties, Hawkeye's included, were in bad shape.

"Mine is dead or nearly dead," Hawkeye decided before huffing off to find Lucky. A younger and slimmer Sloppy Joe, Lucky had arrived two days before and was put in charge of triaging these arrivals. But Lucky looked hopelessly out of his comfort zone, and with a clusterfuck in the making, Hawkeye decided he'd had enough.

"Mine's circling the drain," he announced as he positioned himself equidistant from all four bays and upped the decibels several pips. "Bay 2 is probably unsurvivable. The guy in Bay 1 is tachycardic. Bay 4 needs to go in for a scan right now." Lucky stood back to watch his first assignment go pear shaped and leave a crap first impression. Fernsby, watching Hawkeye reverse-triage the four visitors, turned to Southwark. "If I ever happen to get injured, please don't let him triage me. You owe me at least that much."

9

A Record-Breaking Month

Jock had taken full advantage of his recent find of a small porcelain teapot and some Fortnum & Mason loose-leaf tea. That the tea might have been Southwark's appeared to be of little or no consequence. During the morning meeting, Soleski declared last month to have been a record-breaking one in terms of blood use. With numbers of casualties not significantly different from previous months, it was the clearest indication yet that people were getting increasingly badly injured, fueled by more powerful and often badly contaminated homemade devices.

Hawkeye looked bruised. As he told Southwark over morning coffee, he was given stick for making inappropriate remarks during the morning ward round and told to get with the program. He would like to know who snitched on him, having just returned from Soleski's office after yet another verbal chiding.

"Someone's complained about something I said during the ward round this morning," he told those who feigned interest.

"And so I'm called in for a meeting without coffee, head of the shit parade all because I said that we should stop giving one of the Afghans more opiates as he wouldn't get the same pain meds in any local hospital, so why do it here? Isn't it the whole fucking point that we treat locals only up to the level they can expect to find in Afghanistan, and so why not apply this to meds? Why use epidurals or nerve catheters if we have to take them out anyway at the point of transfer without anything else to put them on?"

Hawkeye seemed to find it difficult to understand why he was singled out when others weren't.

"One of the Americans said about another Afghan that he got what he deserved, and that he's got no arms or legs left so can't dig in any more IEDs. Now how's that a nicer thing to say? And then Fernsby told me that one of the orthopods refused to repair a medial nerve as otherwise the guy could go back to making IEDs and so now he has a hand that doesn't work. And then yesterday during the laparotomy someone joked that we might as well cut the Afghan's nuts off while we're at it so he can't make any more babies. And then I'm the one to get my balls busted."

The controversy around Hawkeye's talk-without-coffee reverberated throughout the Doctors' Room. Should pain relief be continued for this Afghan double amputee and so many others like him? He was on a dose of opiates his local health care system would never in a gazillion years match, and would be discharged within the next few days with nothing stronger than Paracetamol. So why raise his hopes only to throw him off a cliff's edge painwise? The difficulty was that everyone thought it unfair to move him from a sophisticated analgesic to something more humdrum and less effective while still on the ward.

Southwark suggested they wean him off the most powerful opiate twenty-four hours before discharge to ease his reentry into Afghan care, only for his suggestion to be dismissed by one of the nurses. His pain would be so awful, she said, that he would lie howling on the ward, which would be distressing to all the other patients, and to her staff, and so why not give him a handful of

opiates when releasing him to the care of this terrible country just
to carry him over for a couple of days?

"ANYONE TOLD the parents their kid has died?" One of the American nurses popped her head around the door of the Doctors'
Room where Hawkeye, Southwark, Fernsby, and Fellows sat argu-
ing over the merits of organic food. Hawkeye thought the organic
movement part of an elaborate commercial plot. The girl had been
wheeled to the mortuary, kept company by Soleski and a fistful of
paperwork while her parents were still in reception and, impatient
for lack of news, had cornered one of the interpreters, wondering
how their daughter's surgery was getting on, and maybe somebody
should go and tell them?

THE HOSPITAL CORRIDOR smelled yet again of Aunt Jemima this
morning, courtesy of the shrink. Everyone seemed grateful for
small mercies such as breakfast pancakes, peppered eggs, bacon,
beefsteak, and hash browns.

Hawkeye returned from the pre-breakfast ward round red-faced.
One of the surgeons, he said, had not been taken to task over his
remarks about an Afghan casualty when he'd said that the most
likely outcome for one of the insurgents was that he'd go straight
to Guantánamo Bay and get a bullet.

"Has he been reported? I bet you not."

TODAY'S FIRST CASUALTY was a slug through the buttock with a big
exit wound out the front. The casualty, an Afghan male, was rapidly losing blood. Nighy, a freshly arrived anesthetist and Brook's
replacement, told everyone he was having to chase after the Afghan and could they please take their cues from him.

Nighy was in charge of the casualty's physiology—his breathing and blood flow—and drip-fed the surgeons information on

the patient's stability. Problem was that the casualty continued to bleed from an unidentified cavity, and Nighy wasn't able to keep up fluid-wise, he said. Even with blood bags being hand-wrung to up the tempo, the guy was losing blood faster than could be pumped in. Hawkeye ordered him straight into the operating room so as to unzip him sternum to pubis to stem the bleeding.

But Buster and Bomber weren't keen. Was Hawkeye right to think it a major vascular injury that required immediate surgery? Or would a scan show it to be a pelvic injury that only needed washing out? Did Bomber want Hawkeye to be right or wrong? After all, their relationship had never been a happy one. As general surgeons, both spent more time on that razor's edge between life and death than anyone else here. Hawkeye is on his seventeenth tour, Bomber on his eleventh. But then Bomber spent years on the rough side of justice in a violent Mogadishu. These then were the ball-breakers of Bastion: they suffered no incompetence and would not stand for indecision, even if, ironically, their competing viewpoints would occasionally achieve exactly that. Bomber and Hawkeye, so very much alike in so many ways, had plenty reason to give each other a wide berth.

A postoperative scan on the Afghan showed bleeding on the right side of the pelvis, something Hawkeye realized he should have spotted but didn't. Worried by the discovery, Hawkeye was biding his time in the Doctors' Room with the casualty in intensive care biding his when one of the nurses opened the door and looked straight at him.

"You'll want to take a look at this."

"...?"

"It's your patient."

"Well, what about him?"

"You might want to take a look is all."

Hawkeye got up and followed her onto the ICU. He wasn't gone long. Unhappy with the emergency treatment, or if not unhappy then deeply suspicious, Bomber had decided it prudent to finger the Afghan's backside so as to check for internal bleeding, but in doing so had risked decompressing the very belly Hawkeye packed only thirty minutes earlier.

Hawkeye lost no time in seeking out Soleski.

I wondered how Soleski would handle this one. Wondering was what everyone else did too. It is considered bad practice to interfere with another's patient, and particularly so without consulting with the one charged with his care, and Hawkeye was none the happier for Bomber being the miscreant. Bomber would no doubt say he'd been acting in the patient's interest, able to summon Buster's support; after all he was right there when it happened, or so the nurse had said. Nighy told me he thought it all part of Bomber's ploy to find fault with Hawkeye. Their rivalry left Soleski with a difficult choice: to put Bomber and Hawkeye in a room with gloves and let them have it out, or to massage their relationship along as best as he could for however long it might last. As to Hawkeye, Soleski reasoned that protocol meant that casualties were to be taken in for a scan first, and that Hawkeye knew this. Everyone here did. It was the hospital's insurance policy should things go belly-up. And so Soleski went for a sloppy-cock dismissal.

THAT AFTERNOON, all hands were summoned on deck for a US marine whose legs had been blown clear off by yet another roadside bomb. His arms were still attached, even if barely. Brook and Fellows had their work cut out to manage his airway and liquids just to keep him alive. Because he bled so extensively, Hawkeye voiced his view that they take him into the operating room so he could open up the belly and have a look inside. Soleski was quick to overrule: protocol, he reminded everyone, has it that CT takes priority and so into the scanner the lad went, blood product and fluids in tow.

The marine survived. But it required ninety-one pints of blood (by comparison, a healthy adult contains about ten pints of blood), including forty in the scanner alone, and, with hindsight, even Bomber agreed that it would have been better had he been taken straight into theater to gain proximal control. After what happened yesterday, however, no one had any appetite to take on Soleski.

"You can't win, can you?" Hawkeye told Fernsby as he prepared to remove a painful cyst from deep inside the colon of a British soldier, the lad propped up on his knees doggy-style, head twisted sideways, and fast asleep.

"Let's just be happy he survived," Fernsby replied.

I accompanied Hawkeye for some spicy chicken wings at our Pizza Hut–KFC combo outside. We joined three of the female nursing staff around one of the wooden picnic tables.

"Did you see that visiting medic today? Young chap, blond hair, funny Hemingway tash," Hawkeye said to the oldest, whom he'd known from previous tours.

"What about him?"

"Bet right now he's beating off in his sock, eyes closed, and not thinking about you."

"Nor is he thinking about you."

"I bloody well hope not."

THE EVACUATION of casualties is typically performed by one of three helicopter crews: MERT, Dustoff, or Pedro. MERT is a British-staffed medical crew, comprising a physician, one or two advanced paramedics, and an emergency nurse. These operate out of a Chinook, creating what is effectively a mini–emergency room with rotors, and allow for fairly invasive emergency treatment to be given en route, such as blood transfusions, a general anesthetic, and intubation. The crew work in twenty-four-hour shifts—twenty-four hours on, followed by twenty-four on standby—and are located on the flight lines so as to be within running distance of the helicopter. Gunners are positioned to the sides and back of the Chinook, while an RAF crew provide protection and risk their lives in bringing in the casualties. By contrast, Dustoff and Pedro, both named after call signs, are American-staffed helicopter crews that will enter directly into hot zones to collect casualties. Dustoff helicopters fly under the Red Cross and are unarmed. For that reason they are accompanied, as is MERT, by Apache helicopters. Pedro crews, like their Dustoff counterparts, fly straight into active fighting if necessary, two Sikorsky UH-60 Black Hawk helicopters at a time, one to land, the other to provide protection, and are armed. Their crew includes paramedically trained para-rescuemen, or para-rescue jumpers, commonly referred to as PJs. I always felt slightly envious of them as they sauntered in, chalked in yellow desert dust, wild-eyed, casualty in tow, back from the coal face like *Mad Max* characters. These were the adrenaline junkies of the war, and they damn well looked it. Every rescued soldier was handed a challenge coin by the crew, one of a variety, all saying "Saved by Pedro." Hawkeye, having become friendly with one of the PJs, pocketed one too. The level of medical care extended by Dustoff and Pedro is limited, by resource constraint if anything, their primary mission being to deliver a casualty to a field hospital within the golden hour.

An odd sequence of events earlier today brought home both the risk these PJs face and the surreality of this war. Rattled by the experience, I put my thoughts down in an e-mail.

From: Rond Dr M. E. J. de
To: Bud Popsugar
Subject: Couldn't make this stuff up . . .

Dear Bud:

An American gunner has just fallen two hundred feet to his death from his Pave Hawk medevac helicopter, called Pedro, or the American equivalent of MERT. Like our MERT, these Pedros respond to what they here call "9-liners," or structured requests for medical evacuation called in from the ground and, as one might expect, very to the point. . . . Pedro crews (also known as PJs) are pretty hard-core.

The sad irony is that they had been en route to collect a soldier who had fallen fifteen feet from a rooftop and cannot now move his legs.

You couldn't make this stuff up if you tried.

OVER AND ABOVE the usual flutter of wound closures and follow-up procedures, nothing much was afoot today till a boy was ferried in by taxi at dusk. The boy wasn't breathing and had no cardiac output, and his driver claimed to be none the wiser as to how long he had been like that. The injuries didn't rule out the possibility of being hit by a car, quite possibly the taxi, but as usual, truth can be difficult to distinguish from falsehood, and injury trumped truth in any case, and so the resus team began CPR. Hawkeye called for a laparotomy set to be at the ready, seeing that the X-ray showed the belly to be full of liquid. The boy, alas, never so much as made it into the operating room. Time was called. After all, there was no knowing for how long he had already been dead.

With the boy confined to the morgue, and just as our stash of pizzas arrived, five Cat A's were gurneyed in: a double amputee, two GSWs to the abdomen, an Afghan with multiple frags to the face, chest, and abdomen, and one with an injured hand. The pizzas were left to go cold as everyone vacated his bachelor pad and headed for resus. Not sure whether he'd be needed or not, Southwark lingered behind the yellow line. Hawkeye was in scrubs already, as was Fernsby.

"Don't you go start on my pizza," Fernsby told Southwark.

"What'd you order?"

"I'm not telling you."

HAVING SOWN UP two laparotomies, Hawkeye was asked to close the shoulder of a Danish soldier a day earlier than planned. An IED had massacred his Labrador and, in the process, fragged his own shoulder with bits of metal. Dogs are widely used to sniff out explosives, and the Dane had become attached to this one and been given permission to fly home to give her a proper funeral. The dead dog was due out tonight, and the Danish soldier wondered if Hawkeye wouldn't mind closing his wound a day early? But Hawkeye very much minded. He said he had no patience for someone whining over a dog that was to be flown home so it could be chucked in the incinerator there.

"That's far more than they do for their boys here," he told the nurse who relayed the request.

As one nurse wandered off, another came in, oblivious to the exchange that had just taken place. Would Hawkeye please see to a Dane who needs his shoulder closed up?

"No, I bloody well won't! How much more obvious does it need to be that I have no interest in this case? If our boys cannot be flown home when their dad or mum are ill or when their child is being born, why should I care about a fucking Dane who is being repatriated with his mutt? Why not throw the fucking dog on the burn pit with all the legs we've taken off in the last few days?"

She left Hawkeye alone and called on Doo Rag instead.

10

Kandahar

Today was "humpback day" for one of the docs, or the day that marked the midpoint of his six-week tour. Doctors arrived and departed unaccompanied and were, in this as in so many ways, solitary animals. Nurses, by contrast, came and left en masse to give way to a brand-new cohort in a formal handover ceremony before their twenty-four-hour decompression in Cyprus. The mood at their collective departure today was jovial, and when two of the operating room staff were told they could not be accommodated on the same flight back, they took it badly. Camaraderie has always been a strong feature of military life and never more so than in the theater of war. While there is camaraderie among the doctors too, the interpersonal bonds they form are unlikely to be as strong, if only because they deploy for shorter tours, and because their deployments are staggered such that people come and go pretty much every fortnight.

As one of the anesthetists prepared to leave on an evening flight, I felt a pang of jealousy. There was obvious delight on the part of those sallying forth. Nithercott, the gasser, used an anesthetic nerve block, which he inserted and would now monitor, to hitch a medevac flight back to Birmingham. Doing so meant he avoided having to wait for a seat to free up on one of the regular flights back to the UK. He was over the moon, even if his getaway meant piggybacking on an injured infantryman.

I was invited to join one of the docs on a flight to Kandahar to witness the handover of three Afghan casualties to the local health care system. As was customary when moving off base, I suited up in regulation body armor. Aside from two smallish ceramic plates—one at the back, one in the front—my flak jacket provided little protection from the elements—ballistic, explosive, or otherwise, but then again, the chances of getting shot at were relatively small, and, if anything, jackets and helmets were a clammy nuisance in this infernal heat.

The three drop-offs had been strapped to gurneys shackled to the metal floor of a Lockheed C-130 Hercules. For casualty transfers to Lashkar Gah, a short flight away, the Chinook seemed the vehicle of choice. For longer trips, the larger Hercules made for a good trooper for its sheer space and comfort.

Today's casualties were to be dropped off at Kandahar Military Regional Hospital, called Camp Hero,[1] an Afghan National Army forward operating base near Kandahar City. It lies just outside its bigger American sister, itself constructed on the remains of an old and abandoned Soviet base and a bleak reminder of Afghanistan's long courtship with conflict. Camp Hero's fifty-bed hospital is said to be one of the country's best, yet leaves much to be desired in comparison with Camp Bastion's. In practice the Afghan medics, even when asking for advice, often didn't take it, leaving their mentors the ungrateful task of monitoring the money plowed into equipment, supplies, and facilities by the West. At least such was the strong impression left by Weegee's lecture last night on his twelve-month stint at this very hospital.

"They don't even bother to write labels on medications with instructions for use," Weegee told us prior to leaving. "Only one in five ANA soldiers can read, so what's the fucking point?" And whereas antibiotics are thirteen to the dozen, oral opiates are rare as hens' teeth. The irony is of course that plenty of people regularly use opium for their own entertainment—an interesting puzzle for anesthetists, as it can be difficult to know what dose patients are likely to respond to, given the tolerance they've built up over years of opium use.

Chronic prescriptions for officers, Weegee said, are limited to five days—only three for soldiers—meaning that patients have to queue up for the walk-in clinic every few days for meds or even a full course of penicillin. For inpatients, they just leave the injections on the bedside table for the patients or their families to administer. He said that they too use Propofol, not as a continuous drip as in Bastion, but intravenously in small doses using boluses. Problem is, he said, that they only ever do it when the patient begins to move during surgery. And then they only operate thirty hours a week and then not at all from Thursday noon to Saturday morning so as to observe Islamic tradition. It takes one tough cookie to survive in this inferno.

Upon arrival at Kandahar's airfield, the casualties were transferred into American ambulances. My chaperone had made himself comfortable on a jump seat—the only one—in the back. Not wishing to miss out, I wedged my six-foot-two-inch frame bung-like into a small corner. The casualties had been silent throughout the hour-long journey, which was just as well, seeing as there was no interpreter on board. The drivers made a short stop at the American-operated Role 3 hospital before heading for our drop-off point just outside one of the side gates, where a local driver would take receipt of our human cargo. Or that was the idea, in any event. As my chaperone explained, the previous week they'd been kept waiting for three hours in the sun before the driver finally showed up to take the casualties from beyond the US base to the hospital, or a distance of four miles. A suicide bomber detonated just outside these gates not long ago, taking six people with him, and we would not be permitted to venture too far out.

The Afghan driver arrived in an old ambulance, stripped of all its once-useful bits and a ghost of its former self. The driver had no medical training and spoke no English. In the absence of a terp, the handover was managed by frequent gesturing.

"The guy is high on opium," my escort said, having wrestled back one of our oxygen canisters. "These things fetch a fair bit of money on the black market, so we want to hang on to them if at all possible." He crouched down next to the most serious of the three casualties. The man had already been relieved of his 60 percent oxygen supply and was now cut loose from his morphine drip and antibiotics and, despite a bad chest infection, got nothing more than the usual paper-bagged Paracetamol, a peace offering at the feet-end of his gurney.

"In either Lashkar Gah or here you need to be sure to arrive before 1630 or else everyone will have fucked off and these guys are left to fend for themselves. And the first thing these drivers do is to look into the bags to see what drugs we've sent along. Anything morphine goes directly to the driver and never even gets to the patient. And so we leave them here to a slow and painful death. This guy here will die of pneumonia."

My escort, a primary care doctor, said he went to see Hawkeye earlier today as he wanted a second opinion on this third casualty before shipping him off, and wondered what Hawkeye's prognosis was. If you keep him here and treat him, Hawkeye had said, he'll ultimately die. If you take him to Kandahar, he will die too, but a little more quickly. That was all my escort needed to know. And this is what he told an emotional nurse who had been caring for the man. She had initially refused to accompany the casualty to Kandahar—though she ultimately did—and found it difficult to accept the handing over of severely injured locals to what, within the hospital, was widely considered to be a grossly inferior health care provision.

While recovery may never have been in the cards for this particular casualty, the matter of dispatching severely injured locals to their own local hospitals was always sure to generate a reaction from the doctors and nurses, mostly one of exasperation or irritation, never mincing words, though occasionally of anger and sadness too. Perhaps the extent of their outrage is proportionate to the tension, as they experience it, between their dual military and medical obligations. The doctors' medical training might have purged them of some emotional reactions—so as to safeguard "coolness and presence of mind"—but also committed them to always do what's right for the patient, to apply "for the benefit of the sick, all measures which are required," as enshrined in the Hippocratic oath. Yet, at the same time, they were a cog in the military machine, an institution that demanded exclusive and undivided loyalty, and commitment to doing one's duty. Problems arose, of course, when the values of the military and the medical profession came into conflict, and never more so than during these transfers. This conflict was likely to be exacerbated in an environment like Bastion, where like-minded individuals were cut off from wider society for an appreciable amount of time to lead a cloistered way of life, with few if any opportunities to drop the pretense.[2] But the values that embodied the medical profession gave rise to another conflict as well: the principle of compassionate care as against the experience of compassion fatigue. A contemporary adaptation of the Hippocratic oath commits doctors to "remember that . . . warmth, sympathy, and understanding may outweigh

the surgeon's knife or the chemist's drug," reinforcing the importance of compassion and kindness as core values of medical practice. And yet, before long, the ideal gave way to the real as doctors
and nurses tired of compassion and became unable to muster the
sort of sympathy they would have wished to, particularly where
Afghans were concerned.

The flight back to Camp Bastion was a silent one. Among the
passengers were three insurgents, bound and blindfolded, but with
an understanding of English good enough to pick up bits of conversation. Hence we were instructed to keep quiet during the flight
for fear we might accidentally disclose useful bits of information.
Takeoff took much longer than anticipated, seeing that the ramp
at the back of the plane failed to close, leaving no option but to
wait until the equipment decided to cooperate. Then again, no
one seemed too bothered about any of this. And so we gave in
to the relentless perspiring, our breaths short and stale to the
palate. The lads responsible for closing the tailgate stood idly
by meanwhile and, as darkness fell, killed their time and ours
with a hand-shadow puppetry display, using the plane's only
light source to project their childhood fantasies onto the black,
defenseless tarmac.

11

War Is Nasty

Back in Camp Bastion, we caught up with a late fatality: a seven-year-old bilateral amputee. The boy was in bad shape when he arrived, having received fifteen minutes of CPR on the MERT already. Yet they took him in for an emergency laparotomy in any event to cut off any blood supply to the legs so he wouldn't bleed out. Thing is, Fernsby said, he would never have made it. Once the bleeding had been controlled, his stumps were unwrapped to show an injury that was deemed unsurvivable in Afghanistan, and so the decision was made to give him a sufficiently large dose of fentanyl to make sure he'd slip away pain-free. Fernsby complained that the decision should have been made much earlier, as a simple unwrapping of the wounds would have given a good enough prognosis and saved twenty or so minutes of operating.

"It didn't take twenty minutes. I was inside the belly in seven," Hawkeye replied.

"Either way, when he came in he didn't have any blood pressure," Fernsby said.

"But he did have a pulse of 120, and you wouldn't have a pulse if you had no blood."

"Well, I just would have called it earlier is all."

"Right. So when I say I let them die, I'm told I'm wrong. Then I try to not make him die, I'm wrong. Fucking brilliant that is."

In only marginally better shape was another recent arrival: a fifteen-year-old shot in the chest by NATO troops after he failed to heed warning shots, and now a detainee on the ward, guarded twenty-four seven by a US marine.

"How fucking retarded is that?" Hawkeye said. "The boy can't even chinwag with another kid his age, can't go for a pee without a marine watching. Probably didn't even understand what they wanted him to do when they shot him."

NINETEEN HOURS LATER a US marine died on the operating table. It was a miserable way to go, as far as the surgical team was concerned. Dying is bad in any case, but when it happened in the operating room, it stung particularly badly. The casualty had followed the usual route from resus to CT and into the operating theater, in a hospital designed to make every transition as quick and easy as possible. Only about sixty feet separated the lifesaving units. In CT, the doctors tucked in around two computer screens, Southwark squatting, elbow on the table and under his chin, Hawkeye right behind him, and Buster behind Hawkeye, his shoulders too heavy for his frame. Fernsby, Jerrycan, Ty, Jock, Nighy, Weegee, and Sloppy Joe watched in a semicircle, awaiting the verdict. Except for the radiologist formulating his opinion, all were keeping very much to themselves.

The decision was made to operate, and the marine was wheeled into Theater 1, prepped and readied by Smitty and his crew. Fellows took charge of his physiology, assisted by Nighy. Buster and Hawkeye got to work on the chest, opening it up like a clamshell with a cut straight across the chest and just below the nipples and right through the sternum. Jock, Fernsby, Southwark, and Ty looked on, but there was little they could do to help. Runners ferried blood from the adjacent lab in Styrofoam boxes covered by a hard-wearing nylon, two handles on the outer surface, blood and paperwork on the inside, the runners checking, double-checking, and filling in labels even as their colleagues removed the bags for use. Alas, the fairy-tale ending wasn't to be. Despite frenzied efforts to get the marine's heart to circulate blood around the body, it just wouldn't play ball. Fellows called it. It was his first on this tour.

Cold, cynical, and cavalier these surgeons might be, and yet death leaves a pretty damn big footprint. If they were badly affected, so too were the nurses and novices, and Ginger in particular, here on his first tour of duty. As a scrub nurse, he worked closely with the surgeons prior to, and during, procedures. Perioperative nurses like him make sure that the operating theater is set up for the procedure, with the correct equipment to hand, and, post-procedure, that the patient is well enough prepared for transfer to one of the wards.[1] Hawkeye took the twenty-year-old outside for a coffee and a hug to put the world to rights.

"Why do I feel so much worse about this case than others?" Ginger asked him.

"It's probably the totting up of so many deaths. Things just get a bit much and then go bang," Hawkeye replied.

"I saw his birth date: December 1990. Know exactly where I was when he was born. Haven't cried for donkey's years. What the fuck is wrong with me?"

"No one gives a monkey's if you get the waterworks. War is nasty. We all know it is, and we all hate it, and we all deal with it in different ways."

" . . . "

"You just hang in there, cupcake. You're fucking special."

Buster too reeled from the effect of this death. Ordinarily an oasis of calm in Bastion's madhouse, he surprised himself at his own reaction. Why so emotional about this marine when he'd seen so many others go the same way? Was it because he had known all along that operating would be pointless under any circumstances? Was it that he knew, as he later told me, that the guy was beyond help as soon as he arrived, seeing his heart was full but refused to beat, but that he felt that he should give him every possible shot at life, however remote, and take him into theater, but feeling guilty about this because even as he opened the chest he knew that in doing so he was merely going through the motions and that his decision to take him into theater would mean he would die on the operating table and that would be shitty for everyone?

"There's a limit to how many of these tours one can do without becoming immune to the misery," Bomber told me later. He said that here you cannot afford to think that every casualty is someone's most precious possession. Injuries are problems to be solved—no more, no less—and so let's set about solving them as best we can, trying to remain sane in the madness.

WHAT DID NONSTOP exposure to the dead and dying do to people here, I wondered? To witness daily and firsthand death quickened by injury, and to do so time and again, would that not cause even the hardiest and most cynical to wonder at the point of it all, of this war, and of their place in it? Ernest Becker, in his Pulitzer Prize–winning opus, said that the terror of death is our most basic anxiety, and that human behavior can be explained as largely the result of a biological need to control this anxiety. He didn't mince words: "This is the terror: to have emerged from nothing, to have a name, consciousness of self, deep inner feelings, and excruciating inner yearning for life and self-expression—and with all this yet to die."[2]

Becker's bleak take on life is relevant when considering that the twentieth century, for all its progress in medicine, technology, and education, was also the most murderous in recorded history: an estimated 187 million died as a direct result of war, the majority of them civilians.[3] Recent wars in Iraq and Afghanistan involved the deployment of some 2.7 million US troops between 2001 and 2011.[4] As of December 2011, 73 percent of US soldiers had deployed for at least one tour of duty in either war,[5] with 37 percent having deployed at least twice.[6] These numbers do not take into account deployments from the other countries that make up the NATO-controlled ISAF. An estimated 650,000 people lost their lives in these two wars alone,[7] 7,500 of whom were US and UK troops. Data from the UK Ministry of Defense on the Iraq War suggest that the rate of serious to very serious injuries is likely to be as high as 125 percent of this casualty rate. Casualty numbers from other major recent conflicts in Sudan, Libya, Syria, Congo, Gaza, and the Ukraine are less clear, but likely to run into the hundreds of thousands, with the UN estimating 300,000 war-related deaths in the Sudan conflict alone.[8]

In addition to this direct human cost, the psychological costs of war are becoming ever more apparent. Incidence of post-traumatic stress disorder (PTSD) among military personnel is significantly higher than among the general population: up to 31 percent lifetime rates in the United States, compared with around 5 percent for the general population. Active-duty suicides among US troops reached an all-time record of 349 in 2012, exceeding US combat deaths that year. Even if correlation need not mean causation, the US Department of Veterans Affairs reported that in 2009 the suicide rate among veterans was double that of the general population. Similarly, of the 220,000 British troops deployed between 2001 and 2014, around 27 percent are estimated to develop a mental health issue at some point. The UK charity Combat Stress reported a 26 percent increase in referrals among ex–service personnel for treatment of PTSD, in 2014.[9] While such related concepts as "shell shock" and "irritable heart" have been around since the First World War, PTSD was only recognized as a distinct category by the American Psychiatric Association in 1980, to signal a change in the acceptance of psychological injury.[10] Prior to this, psychological injury was stigmatized and considered a form of disgrace to the soldier. Such was the stigma that in the post-1945 period, admissions registers and case notes for officers who had been treated for psychological disorders were systematically destroyed to protect the patient's identity.[11] Psychiatrists were unflatteringly referred to as "shrinks," "trick-cyclists," and "nut-pickers."

According to the US Department of Veterans Affairs (2015), 20 to 30 percent of those who served in Iraq and/or Afghanistan show symptoms of PTSD. In the UK, a survey of 9,990 UK veterans placed PTSD prevalence at 4 percent, with common mental disorders, including depression and anxiety, at 19.7 percent and alcohol misuse at 13 percent.[12] It is not clear why UK forces have consistently been found to appear to "fare better" than their US counterparts over the past twenty years. It might be owing to differences in measurement or definition, as non-US psychiatrists tend to rely on the World Health Organization's ICD-10 criteria rather than the DSM-5 used by the American Psychiatric Association,[13] to US service personnel being younger on average and of a lower socioeconomic background than their British counterparts, and to much longer average deployment durations for US forces.[14]

Data on psychological injury among medical personnel at war is harder to come by because medics in general are understudied as compared with other emergency and rescue personnel when it comes to psychological injury.[15] One study of British military health professionals estimated 35 percent to suffer psychological injury,[16] while another found the rate of psychological injury to be equivalent to that of deployed nonmedical military staff.[17] This particular study also found no significant difference when comparing rear-located medics with those actually facing combat. One explanation for the comparatively high incidence of psychological injury among military medics—even taking into account their training, experience, and noncombat role—is that they are typically assembled in groups only weeks before their deployment, as compared with combat units who might spend up to a year training together.[18] This is relevant in that high morale and good interpersonal relationships in a team have been found to provide some protection against serious adverse reactions to traumatic experiences.[19]

That exposure to the consequences of war was experienced as personally traumatic by the surgical staff seems evident from the coping responses found in Camp Bastion. These responses appear to fall into two general camps: attempts to escape the real, and attempts to recover what was lost.

"Avoidance coping" and "escape coping" are well-known mechanisms by means of which people dodge having to deal with a particular stressor in an attempt to protect themselves from psychological anguish.[20] Each Wednesday night, for example, was marked by a repatriation service that all troops stationed in Camp Bastion, including hospital staff, were expected to attend. It was here that fallen NATO troops were remembered before being sent home for burial. Many would have arrived already dead at the hospital; a few would have died in resus; only occasionally would people die on the operating table. Even so, several of the docs took pains to avoid attending the service—by, for instance, asking colleagues to page them en route so as to have an excuse to be elsewhere. And while they might be expected to have a professional interest in checking up on their patients during quiet times, it was rare to see a surgeon on the wards outside of the required twice-daily rounds. These ward rounds were a frequent source of complaint by the ward nurses, who thought them noisy and unruly, with doctors paying little attention to patients other than those they were expected to give an opinion on and regularly needing to be called to attention. This lack of engagement with the still living, and the dead, appears to reflect an attempt to avoid reconnecting with those at the prickly end of conflict. What is interesting is that doctors' attempts to avoid emotional engagement coincided with their worry and guilt about not being more deeply affected emotionally by what they bore daily witness to. They thus actively avoided becoming emotionally engaged even as doing so left them guilt-ridden.

A different form of avoidance is the bracketing of experience, where both damage-control resuscitation and surgical staff would consider their deployment as a temporary state of affairs and as different from the normality to which they would soon return. They hoped to contain the experience of war by framing it as the exception to the rule—the rule being "the everyday" back home—and as temporary. That way, their experience needn't bleed into, or otherwise affect, life back home. And it may partly be due to this desire for compartmentalization as a coping mechanism that returning medics are often reluctant to speak openly about their experiences of war except, of course, with each other. Or their silence can be explained by their reluctance to revisit the darkness that resides not outside, but inside. War correspondent Chris Hedges wrote that "fundamental questions about the meaning, or meaninglessness, of our place on the planet are laid bare when we watch those around us sink to the lowest depths. War exposes the capacity for evil that lurks not far below the surface within all of us."[21] This darkness arises not just out of the selfishness and lack of regard for others that war exposes, but also out of the pleasure we experience at inflicting cruelty and death, and the adrenaline highs that accompany war.

Aside from attempts to escape the real, there were also plenty of attempts at recovering what they had lost. This coping mechanism is designed to recover some sense of familiarity so as to counter experiences of surreality, and also to recover some sense of control so as to counter experiences of futility. For example, such routines as pizza night Fridays and pancake breakfast Sundays appear to have been invented, or imported, by the doctors so as to try to establish enclaves of normality, familiarity, and home comfort. This is noteworthy in part because, in Camp Bastion's hospital, as in the theater of war more broadly, there is no real distinction between weekdays and weekends—one is always "on"—except the idea of a weekend "imposed" by pizzas and pancakes. The near beer was always in plentiful supply, something surgeons and anesthetists would enjoy in the evening, much like one might relax over real beer in a bar or pub after work. There were poker evenings and sports days. Home comforts were valued commodities, shared, and typically arrived in packages sent from home. These packages included such things as newspaper articles, crossword puzzles, magazines, colorful and handmade surgical hats, candies, and homemade shortbread. The Doctors' Room had a computer and provided constant and reliable access to the Internet, meaning that surgeons and anesthetists took turns updating their Facebook profile and replying to e-mails, and generally kept up social-media-wise. None of this was formally organized or sponsored by the military organization; these collective initiatives were intended to provide some sense of normalcy and rhythm to an otherwise relatively austere and alien environment.

Even the Estonian contingent, which included two surgeons, an anesthetist, and a nurse, had their own enclaves of normality. They lived in a small fenced-off enclosure within Camp Bastion, equipped with its own sauna (in a desert where temperatures would regularly exceed 113 degrees Fahrenheit, or 45 degrees Celsius, in summer).

The irony of course is that attempts at reclaiming the familiar may, paradoxically, have served as reminders of the absurdity of the human condition in the context of Afghanistan's war. If anything, the availability of home comforts made the environment even more surreal: real battle helicopters taking off as surgeons watched the helicopter scene in *Apocalypse Now*; a sauna in the desert; a KFC–Pizza Hut; the Easter Bunny walking past an incinerator. At best, then, bringing in home comforts, such as in the avoidance strategies described above, offered a temporary escape from, instead of a resolution of, the lived experience of war.

A final set of coping mechanisms appears to have been designed to reequip oneself with a sense of being in control of one's destination. Feelings of being in control can be difficult to sustain amid the lack of privacy, the unpredictability of casualty arrivals, and the sense of futility that characterize the lived experience of war. The attempt to regain some sense of agency might explain why doctors went to great lengths to create private spaces (by draping linens, flags, towels over bits of wire strung around their sleeping quarters) or to grow flowers and vegetables in the desert. The former would be consistent with observations made elsewhere that territorial strategies form an important means of controlling the absurd circumstances of life,[22] the latter with gaining control in the face of the felt futility of work at war by cultivating an otherwise trivial patch of fertile soil on the patio behind the Doctors' Room. In similar fashion, a group of trauma surgeons deployed during 2012–13 decided to try to bake their own bread, using a sourdough starter brought to Bastion from Devon, England. They used the camp's kitchens, during lulls in the afternoon, to bake their bread and proceeded to share it around. The warmth and freshness of the bread, particularly when in time for afternoon tea, drew a sharp contrast with the experience of the dead and dying, and was consciously intended as a counterpoint to "the bloody routine of daily life [at war]":

> As in the series MASH, the counterpoint to the tales of blood, heroism, and medical miracles was the humour and the humanity that punctuated the bloody routine of daily life; but, instead of a potato distillery brewing alcohol, we made bread. . . . In the end, the legacy of this club of five military consultants—an emergency physician, a US general surgeon, a paediatric surgeon, and two anaesthetists—is embodied in their Bastion tour T shirt: "Make bread not war."[23]

"Make bread not war" symbolized defiance. Other examples might include refusals to engage with "trivial" cases such as an Afghan with persistent pain in his bowel and erection problems, and a request to close a Danish soldier's shoulder one day early so he could accompany his dead dog on its flight home. It is doubtful that such attempts to reclaim a sense of control were able to resolve the sense of futility that often characterized the lived experience of war, and which persisted regardless of these efforts. At best they might have offered a temporary escape from the debilitating feeling of being involved in something futile, introducing a degree of personal excitement that temporarily punctuated the boredom and monotony of daily life at Camp Bastion.[24]

12

Way to Start Your Day

Rarely did a morning or evening pass without its predictable delivery of human cargo, typically soldiers with limb injuries so severe that they required amputation. Unusually, this morning's first arrivals were children and an adult, four in all, presumed to be members of the same family. The kids had stumbled on an explosive while playing outside. Sloppy Joe strapped on a lead apron as he readied himself for their arrival. Such aprons were worn by all gathered around the trauma call to help protect against harmful X-rays fired by a portable machine wheeled in as part of the primary survey. Joe had an Operation Vampire on his hands, meaning at least one of the kids had needed an emergency blood supply during the short flight to Camp Bastion. The medical team on board the Chinook carries a cool box supplied with blood to cater to different blood types to prevent casualties bleeding out. By the time the helicopter touched ground, one of the children had already expired. It quickly emerged that one of the surviving two had a big hole in his head and was missing both eyeballs. His brain tissue was visible through the gap and, as he was logrolled, began to bleed into an empty socket.

"Is he dead yet?" Southwark asked.

"Not yet. Won't be long," Hawkeye said.

"What about the others?"

"Second kid's being scanned. Brain's fucked."

"And the girl?"

"Her brain's fucked as well."

"I think that's their father there."

". . ."

"Hell of a way to start your day."

None of the three kids ever so much as made it into the operating room. The injured adult was screened off to protect him from the worst as monitors and anesthetic equipment were switched off and tubes and sensors withdrawn. By 0900, several other relatives had arrived and been seated in reception, given a terp and various sets of papers to fill out in duplicate as the threesome prematurely slipped into the chilly netherworld of Bastion's morgue, to be released into their family's care later in the day.

WHEN ENTERING resus from DFAC after a Wheaties and Coco Pops breakfast washed down with instant coffee, Fernsby and I wandered into a waft of freshly fried bacon, its source soon obvious: two badly burned Afghans occupied opposite tables, attended to by emergency staff. The first registered at 53 percent burns, the second at 48 percent, both readings the result of a standard calculation using the "rule of nine": divide the body in multiples of nine, with the head, chest, and abdomen accounting for 9 percent each if completely burned, the back and buttocks for 18 percent, 9 percent for each arm and 18 percent for each leg, 9 percent for the front, 9 percent for the back. Anything over 35 percent isn't normally considered survivable in Afghanistan, or so Jock had told me earlier, so such patients are given palliative care from the word go. The first of the two died within the hour. The second would follow soon after but insisted on seeing a terp meanwhile, who in turn motioned for Hawkeye to come over for no good reason other than that he happened to be walking past.

"He says he thinks he's dying," the terp said.

"He is," Hawkeye replied.

"He wants you to take him and his friend back to the valley where the helicopter found them."

"His friend's dead."

"   "
. . .

"   "
. . .

"Yes he says he knows. He wants you to organize a car to take them both back."

"Right. So where does he think we're going to get a taxi from?"

"   "
. . .

"Tell 'em we will see what we can do," Fernsby, who had joined the conversation, said to the terp, who told the Afghan, who slowly moved his blackened hand over his left upper chest and looked grateful.

Fernsby wandered off in the direction of the administrative wing of the hospital to find Soleski and sort out transport. Southwark, Buster, and Hawkeye repaired to the Doctors' Room for a dose of *Jackass** to help lift the spirits. Hawkeye, famished from not having eaten anything all day, found himself a cold slice of beef, smuggled in from our American friends next door, and had it down in no time.

A COUPLE OF US marines arrived by Pedro around midday, with relatively minor injuries. One had a gunshot wound to the upper leg, the other a slug fragment in his right cheek. They made for a

---

* The MTV reality series.

lively pair, sky-high on adrenaline after a gunfight with the Taliban. One boasted he had shot and killed six Taliban before being hit himself with a fragment that, as far as he could tell, had ricocheted off his helmet or one of the vehicles and buried itself in his face. His friend in the next bay over promptly killed the insurgent before being shot in the leg himself.

The remainder of the day was quiet until a man with a hole in his head returned a good forty-eight hours earlier than anticipated from a rendezvous with Kandahar's neurosurgeon. Having first arrived in Bastion yesterday, he was flown out and back again within a twelve-hour window. Problem was that the surgical team in Kandahar forgot to send along the two-square-inch bit of skull-back they'd removed to relieve the pressure of blood against his brain. Ordinarily this would have been stitched into a specially created pocket just underneath the skin of the abdomen. Yet there was no trace of any incision anywhere except the ritual circumcision and bolt hole in his head. Suspicions were that Kandahar discharged the wrong head injury. Meanwhile, the Afghan had set up shop in intensive care, looking around unsteadily, clearly unaware of the soup sandwich he had become thanks to a sloppy handover. His missing piece presumably lay wrapped in cellophane somewhere in Kandahar, ready for dispatch.

At the onset of sunset, and just as Sloppy Joe called for volunteers to help him lug around the weekly pile of pizzas, a motley band of pagers heralded the arrival of a Cat A. The whiteboard listed it as a US marine who'd been hit by a rocket-propelled grenade. While Hawkeye, Nighy, and Fernsby headed for resus, I offered to meet Sloppy Joe and Southwark in five, or as soon as they'd had a quick look in. We made our way from reception into the black hot night to where the light pollution was, signposting the makeshift square with its crude KFC–Pizza Hut combo, NAAFI, and games room.

A short queue had already formed at the shipping container's window. The scent they gave off was unmistakable, evoking a lazy day out topped off with fast food and soda and feet-up television. Stacked up on one of the two ovens were twenty-one pizzas, hot to the touch, though there's always a risk they'll be stone cold by the time the casualty is dispatched with. To my surprise, this happened more quickly than I expected.

"Casualty's a hero," Joe said.

"Right," I replied. "Gone to Camp Hero."

"He *is* a hero."

". . ."

"The guy is dead."

". . ."

It was right about then and there that I became aware of a nauseating feeling ascending from my gut: a rotten-to-the-core sense of relief, less at a merciful end to years of pain and rehabilitation than at the prospect of hot pizza and companionship. The sense of shame I felt then I've not felt since. After all, what was a pizza compared with the life of a soldier? What the fuck was wrong with me?

We sat down to watch *Lock, Stock and Two Smoking Barrels.*

OUR HOLE-IN-THE-HEAD caught up with his skullcap the following morning. It arrived as a stowaway on a midnight flight from Kandahar, wrapped in cling film and with a Post-it Note. One of the orthopods had been asleep on the sofa when the keep-safe arrived. At a loss as to what to do with it, and keen to be reunited with the sofa, he stuck it in our small fridge, figuring it as good a place as any. At least it would keep until morning. And there it remained until ten o'clock, next to our soda pop, near beer, and Maltesers. Ty, meanwhile, was busily rooting through various drawers, nooks, and crannies in the Doctors' Room.

"What are you hoping to find?" Fernsby asked him.

"An electric toothbrush," Ty said.

"What for?"

"To cross-pollinate my tomatoes."

"..."

"There's no bees out here so I've got to do it myself." Ty's private obsession with growing tomatoes in the desert seemed to have provided him with a distraction from the humdrum of hospital life. It was his way of sticking up two fingers to this desolate and death-ridden Helmand hellhole.

"Wouldn't a Q-tip be simpler? Should have some in primary care, I would have thought."

FIVE BLEEPERS SANG in unison. Three Cat A's en route to Bastion: a GSW wound to the head, one to the buttock, and one to the arm. All three were infantry. Word on the ground was that it was another "green on blue" insofar as a member of the Afghan National Army working alongside the boys had turned on them, taking potshots.

Hawkeye was given the buttock to deal with. The soldier told him it had felt as if someone had thrown a stone against his backside in a teasing sort of way, and so he turned around expecting a smirk but instead saw his friend on the ground and another mate clutching his arm. And he then realized they had been shot, as had he.

"Shot in me fuckin' arse," he said, "so now I've got another hole for them to go into."

With morphine taking the edge off the pain, and with the wound given the all clear for operating, Hawkeye and the infantryman were left to kill time while one of the anesthetists got himself ready to take over the guy's breathing.

"The Afghan National Army are the gayest people I've ever met," the infantryman continued. "Did you know that the Pashto have seven different words for gay: for those who receive it, give it, the little fun boy who gets it whenever anyone wants it . . ."

With that he was out, four short of his tally, his bare flesh quickly exposed.

"Another success story," Hawkeye said.

"Yup . . . integration is working well, isn't it?" Nighy replied.

"SCOUSE'S BACK," I told Hawkeye. Scouse had been on our OPTEC course in Portsmouth just prior to being flown out to one of the forward operating bases to take over from an injured colleague. He was a physician from Liverpool, had recently married, and had seemed anxious about his imminent departure.

"He's here for a couple of days till he can get a flight out. Lucky bastard is on R&R." Military staff who deploy for periods longer than the hospital doctors' typical six-week tour get a two-week break "rest and recuperation" and are flown home to reconnect with family and friends, even if their closest pals are those left behind in Afghanistan's poppy fields.

"Don't see the point of R&R, frankly," Fernsby said. "By the time you get used to being back home it is time to come back. And while you're home all you want is to be back with your mates."

"He's had a boring tour so far. Only one shot fired, at a dog, and that one ricocheted off a compound wall and hit a villager instead," said Hawkeye.

"Imagine that went down brilliantly," Fernsby said.

"Minor injury apparently. But the village was pretty pissed off about the whole thing."

" . . ."

"You should ask Scouse to tell you about his last tour here. He has this great story about when they had entered some compound and got surprised by a suicide bomber who ran up to them and blew himself to smithereens. Thing is, it didn't go quite as planned and only part of the explosive went off, and so instead of flinging outwards it shot the guy's head right up in the air like a fucking champagne cork."

"   "

"I'm still not sure about these ragheads," said Hawkeye, as he eyed a handful of Afghans sauntering around the hospital. "People like that used to have to queue up for twenty-four hours outside the gate before being allowed to sell their wares in the camp, and now they're here permanently. None of these trinket shops was here on my last tour. How the fuck do we know that they're not plotting against us?"

"The terps seem okay to me," Fernsby said.

"Just saying you can never be sure."

TOILET PAPER DOUBLED up as coffee filter as I prepared the docs a brew and put on the kettle for tea. Sky News strutted its trophy stories on the telly in the background. Its overnight haul excited no one but their anchor, and how could it in this microcosm of brutality? Doctors wandered in and out for a post-breakfast lift-me-up before the morning meeting of departments and, beyond that, a short list of electives.

As Southwark cranked up the volume on the TV set, several bleepers went off simultaneously.

"Cat A. Five minutes," Fellows told me as he joined a handful of surgeons heading like wildebeests for resus down the corridor and to the right. Not ten minutes later they were back in their seats. Hawkeye, last in, sliced two fingers across his throat.

"UK, US, or Afghan?"

"UK Rifles."

They sunk back into the spots they had vacated only moments ago, to resume their involuntary stupor, only to be told that another fresh hail of casualties was on its way: a gunshot wound to the neck, a gunshot wound to the thigh, and yet another unlucky victor in the roadside bomb lottery. A further three had suffered minor injuries but came along for the ride and would be here shortly.

"What the fuck is Doo Rag in resus for?" Hawkeye said to no one in particular but loud enough for all to hear. "He's booked himself in for all the electives and now trying to get a bite of the casualties too. And why is Buster all over the neck injury when I'm meant to be doctor one for today? I can tell you why. It's because he's Buster, and because he can. Yesterday I was doctor fucking forty-three and the day before fifty-six and the day before that one-hundred-and-thirty-three and tomorrow four-hundred-and-ten and today supposedly doctor number one but not really number one. How the fuck's that right?"

Southwark and Fernsby, in the meantime, were taking bets (to be paid off in pizza purchases) on whether the incoming amputee would turn out to be a single or double, left or right leg.

"A pepperoni on the left," Southwark said.

"I'd say a double. If it is you're buying Friday," Fernsby replied.

AT 1734, A THIRTEEN-YEAR-OLD from one of the forward operating bases was wheeled in. He'd had emergency surgery on his chest already, and both legs had been amputated, but there was more work to be done on his arm and face. The original plan had been to drop him off at Kandahar's American hospital to see the ophthalmologist, but, as Soleski said, when they phoned the hospital the eye specialist was nowhere to be found, and they were reluctant to accept a casualty in his absence, so could they please drop him off at Bastion instead?

Kandahar wasn't exactly flavor of the month. One of the anesthetists returned from there earlier today after handing over a GSW to the jaw for specialist treatment, only to be told that the same Afghan he just dropped off was ready for collection and could he please get a move on? Ordinarily that would have been fine, he said, except that nothing whatsoever had been done to fix the injury.

"This kind of stuff is so bloody frustrating," he had said. "I've been screaming inside my head for years. I don't mind making the trips so long as they have a purpose, but this has clearly been a massive waste of resources."

He slugged his way over to the airfield. Three Americans meanwhile had turned up at the hospital with minor frag wounds. One of them lay on his gurney bellowing "The Star-Spangled Banner" as if without a care in the world. All three should return to the front lines after one or two good nights of recuperation on the ward. A fourth American was diagnosed as suicidal and shipped back to the United States.

A fifth American was less fortunate, the lion's share of his legs having been minced after tripping a wire. Ferried in at just after 2200, he was placed in the care of Cold Feet, with Doo Rag, Hawkeye, Southwark, Jerrycan, and Fernsby as attending surgeons.

"He is still awake," Hawkeye hissed at Ty as both scrubbed at the sink.

"Fucking hell. You mean Cold Feet's not anesthetized him yet?"

"I mean he hasn't gone off to sleep yet and so now he's moving about as they're taking his legs off. What the fuck do they send a klutz like him to a place like this for?"

"We've been thinking," Hawkeye said, "that maybe you could trade two or three of these medical clowns around here for somebody who can find his way around the pulmonary anatomy when the bases are loaded . . ."

"And it's the ninth inning," Duke said.

"Listen," Henry said. "I'll give it to you just the way the General would give it to you. Do you guys think this is Walter Reed? You're doing fine."

"We are like hell," Hawkeye said. "We're swinging with our eyes closed, and . . ."

". . . and up to now we've just been lucky," Duke said.

"Forget it," Henry said. "How's the beer?"[1]

HAWKEYE WAS AWOKEN at a few minutes past midnight and again at 0400 and asked to make his way to the hospital as new casualties were on their way. The first turned out to be a false alarm but not until Hawkeye had legged it to resus. The four o'clock wasn't. Two local women had arrived with bullet holes in their legs. Someone who identified himself as a brother stood idly by, insisting, as they did too, that they be treated by a female attendant. Weegee, the attending emergency department coordinator, ignored the request, saying they have no such luxury in Afghan hospitals so why give them that option here?

After a quiet day, at around 1900, nine casualties arrived within thirty minutes of each other, including five girls with gunshot wounds: two to the chest, the rest through the arms, legs, and belly. The girls had long eyelashes and olive complexions, their hands covered in henna tattoos. There wasn't a tear in sight. The emergency and surgical teams were brilliant to watch. When the proverbial hit the fan, they salvaged what war destroyed, giddy for being productive. The curse in Bastion was never that of too much work but rather the insufficiency of it. Once the casualties had received emergency treatment, and the surgeons had repaired for near beers in the Doctors' Room, it turned out the girls might have been shot by our own helicopters in error. Their thirty-millimeter cannon rounds were designed to fragment upon impact such that anyone within ten meters of an exploding round risked serious injury, and tonight's GSWs looked far more like fragments, the docs said, than the usual bullets.

WHEN I WOKE UP this morning I had no inkling that today was to be my last in Camp Bastion. The final date of my tour had always been up in the air, as it was for many, for the simple reason that everything hinges on the availability of seats on the flight home. These are allocated in order of priority, and neither Hawkeye nor I would have ranked anywhere near the top of the waiting list, even if, for all intents and purposes, our tour was over. The alternative to flying back on a scheduled flight was to join a medical evacuation by assisting the onboard medical team or, in my case, being allowed to observe a medevac team at work during the seven-or-so-hour flight back to Birmingham, UK. It is there that casualties were transferred to Queen Elizabeth Hospital for further treatment. These flights left Helmand in the evening to arrive at around 0300 in Birmingham, where an ambulance would be waiting. What remained from then on was a short journey through a sleeping city to the intensive care unit. The casualties, many of whom would have been anesthetized prior to evacuation, would wake up on home soil with few, if any, memories of their time in Camp Bastion except those triggered by handwritten comments, always encouraging, by nurses in a notebook designed for just that purpose. There was a medevac flight out tonight, and did I want to be on it?

I conducted a couple of final interviews and said my good-byes. As I readied my kit to fly back, I couldn't help but feel guilty for not being more emotional about it all. In some ways it seemed right to try to reciprocate emotionally the Charlie Foxtrot that looked back at you in turn, often without hope or expectation or indeed any understanding of why they had to be at the shitty end of mankind's cruelty.

13

Back Home

When packing for my return journey, I left behind almost all my clothes—they felt dirty, contaminated—conscious that I might somehow transport the experience back home. I never did pick up my last muslin of laundry. I left my Crocs in the changing room adjacent to the theaters for others to use, but mostly because they had sauntered through the blood of so many casualties.

I looked in on the infantryman whose number had finally come up during this morning's patrol. He would be my ticket home, and I couldn't help but feel embarrassed for being appreciative.

As I readied myself for the medevac flight, I felt guilty for not being more deeply affected emotionally by what I'd seen. I realized that I'd stopped dreaming. I couldn't do God no more. I wasn't able to get it up. I felt tainted by the suffering of others and unable to shake the sensation of voyeurism: of intruding on private suffering with nothing whatsoever to offer in return. My scholarly ambitions jarred badly with the life-and-death scenarios faced by these doctors, and served as a reminder of the spinelessness of much of what we flog off as scholarship. Even at the best of times, my own academic work compared poorly to the most mundane of medical interventions here. I was keenly aware of being able to beat a retreat at any time to grab something to eat, to catch up on sleep, or simply to recharge, without reason or explanation, an extravagance not parceled out to the doctors and their patients. The headwork was exhausting. I returned home intolerant of bullshit. I wrote Hawkeye a note:

From: Rond Dr M. E. J. de
To: Hawkeye
Subject: back home

I am about to hang myself from boredom. And what worries me more than boredom is that I don't seem to be more affected by the trauma in Bastion. I never saw injuries as bad, nor cases as sad, as the young lads and kids whose lives will now be forever changed by no choice of their own. I occasionally need to pinch myself to realize it was for real and am desperately keen not to forget—both in fairness to those affected and in the hope that I might become a better person as a result. How do you deal with all this stuff? With the emotion (or perhaps non-emotion) of it all?

He wrote back straightaway:

From: Hawkeye
To: Rond Dr M. E. J. de
Subject: Re: back home

Don't feel any guilt about not feeling emotion. If we got emotional about what we have just done or seen we would never be able to do it again or live with ourselves. When I got back I spoke at length with the parents of the double amputee with no balls—that was probably the hardest bit of the whole tour! They asked such direct and relevant questions about what happened, what we did, why we did it, did he suffer? etc. Through the Mum, Dad asked if he had a willy (knowing he had no balls). I simply said that I pushed my rubber tube down something that had to be his willy—they laughed . . . how strange, as we all know he still may die.

Even today, five years later, I still feel a lingering impatience with all things trivial. If we, social scientists, took stock of the problems we have solved to date, and their consequences for humanity, would we have reason to be proud? Where are the *real* problems that should guide our research? We know the world is complex and that our knowledge of it is imprecise and incomplete, and so where is that point beyond which we profess to know and, based on this, to act? When did we ever stop human suffering on such scales as witnessed in Iraq and Afghanistan—or on any scale, for that matter? What did we ever do to stop this or any war?[1]

I am ashamed to admit that, like many, I miss the adrenaline-fueled world of combat surgery and the trough of sorrow and indignity into which we dip and by which we are stained for, upon inspection, we find that we have soiled ourselves.

So why is it that the smarting of others enchants us humans so? We have, Edmund Burke wrote, "a degree of delight, and that no small one, in the real misfortunes and pains of others."[2] Anthony Loyd told of his dual addiction to war and heroin, Karl Marlantes of his pleasure at doing battle, likening it to crack cocaine and wondering why a good and decent person like him could love something that hurt people so much. Field Marshal William Joseph Slim said how one of his personal kills, while brutal, gave him "a feeling of the most intense satisfaction."[3] Hemingway wrote of the experience of hunting man as some do of taking heroin: "Those who have hunted armed men long enough and liked it never care for anything else thereafter."[4]

A US Army soldier recalled laughing at a man whose leg had been shot clear off, and how the man kept crawling around until he crawled no more, and thinking to himself, "That was a fucking human being, you son of a bitch. You fucking crazy bastard, that was a human being you fucking killed." And yet, he'd do the same thing again, he said, for "it's like an evil thing inside your body."[5] To a monster, everyone is a monster,[6] and when veterans don't talk about war perhaps it isn't because they suspect we won't appreciate its horrors, but because we won't understand its pleasures.

While the doctors and nurses featured here are not typically exposed to the thrill of the fight, they are willing spectators nonetheless to all that war destroys. Theirs are the best seats in the house to a massacre that repels and intoxicates, a spectacle that flaunts humankind's best and worst in never quite equal measure.

"The human heart dares not stay away too long from that which hurt it most," the American novelist Lillian Smith wrote. "There is a return journey to anguish that few of us are released from making."[7] The ordinary no longer quenches one's thirst, and I'm pained by the realization that my fate as ethnographer is perhaps not so different after all from that of the soldier, surgeon, and war correspondent, in that our pleasure is proportionate to another's pain.

Epilogue

You weren't supposed to read this.

The idea of writing something that would bring the lived experience of doctors at war closer to the general public was originally that of a high-ranking medical officer (whom I'll refer to as the Officer from now on). He had been instrumental in helping to secure permission for my deployment to Afghanistan. My initial hopes were no more ambitious than to produce one or two scholarly articles based on the fieldwork. The Officer had read one of my previous books, *The Last Amateurs*, and was keenly aware that no such work existed on rear-located medical staff. Could I be persuaded to write a similar book about them? Given that he was a veteran of many tours and well versed in the contemporary literature on war, I considered myself in good hands, and what began as a suggestion—one that I wasn't opposed to but had not seriously considered until he raised the possibility—became resolve: over the next couple of years I was to receive more than twenty e-mails, and about the same number of text messages, to remind me specifically of our project. Here are some examples:

I do think the whole military team issue is ripe for a "last amateurs" type book. Thoughts?

Upon my return from Camp Bastion, and again with reference to my rowing ethnography:

Mark

Hope CCAST flight was useful- pse give me a call when you are rested and we can discuss your thoughts about the whole experience.

There are lots of parallels with the "last amateurs" I think; although the conflict is still ongoing you joined a particular group in their own race preparation and saw them out on the ground

And ten days later:

Any more thoughts on the "last bastion amateurs" project?

As if I needed reassurance that, like *The Last Amateurs*, it did not need to be a scholarly text but one that would speak to the general public:

The "last bastion amateurs" is a distinct project to your academic study.

I had promised, upon my return, to write a report for the surgeon general on my observations of teamwork during my deployment. This report included detailed descriptions of examples of the consequences of boredom, of the lack of psychological safety, and of the experience of futility among medical staff. The Officer perused a draft of it and wrote

Mark

Excellent—the vignettes are v strong—the basis of a book!!!

To be confronted daily with the human consequences of war had left me feeling disillusioned with what I felt was a pedestrian, low-stakes, egocentric game of academia. For a while afterward I toyed with the idea of abandoning my academic post at Cambridge and retrain as a surgeon instead:

Mark
    Never too old for med school; but in the first place tell our story with the book!

As I began drafting the book based on my field notes, I became aware that some of the material, upon reading, might not curry favor with the Ministry of Defence. When I shared my reservations about some of the material with the Officer, worrying that not all of it would make for comfortable reading, he dismissed my concerns, insisting that I write candidly and without fear of censorship. He sent me a link to a piece in the *Spectator* magazine, by Tony Harnden, that told of how the MoD were so keen to prevent his own book, *Dead Men Risen*, from publication that they bought, and pulped, the entire print run at a cost of £151,450 to the British taxpayer.

Unlike me, Harnden had signed "an inch-thick contract" agreeing to submit any book manuscript to the Ministry of Defence for it to be checked for "operational security" and "accuracy." The review process that ensued "felt like the literary equivalent of undergoing several colonoscopies a week," Harnden wrote, and resulted in requests for 493 changes to be made. Many of these changes were inconsequential and designed to burnish the reputations of certain officers. Threats of an injunction and DA Notice later,[1] the ministry finally dropped the matter but not before deleting a notable clause in their settlement with Harnden, namely to deal with the publisher and author "on a fair and transparent basis" in the future. As Harnden wrote, there was at least some honesty and consistency in that. His excellent article is worthwhile reading in full.[2]

I wondered as to the Officer's intentions in sending me a link to the Harnden article. Should I worry, I inquired, upon which he replied:

No—just educational . . .

There was quite clearly a sense that a candid account of the everyday experience of combat surgical teams would be a welcome addition to the war literature. This was also my impression from others during my deployment in Camp Bastion, and indeed my field notes contain several references to discussions with Hawkeye and others about the idea of writing a book about their experience of war. I had left a copy of *The Last Amateurs* in the Doctors' Room for anyone to pick up and read, which several did, and which they commented on and appeared to have enjoyed.

I finished a thinly disguised first draft in December 2012. The Officer meanwhile was on his own tour of duty to Camp Bastion and asked to read a copy of it. I explained that I could only ever show him the text on the explicit understanding that this would be for his eyes only, and not to be passed on in any way, shape, or form. With a written promise of confidentiality under my belt, I sent him the work-in-progress. The Officer read the draft, expressed concern and, without further consultation, sent the confidential manuscript straight on to the office of the surgeon general, who made a beeline for my vice chancellor. He wished to discuss what I could, and could not, write about. The vice chancellor's office passed the baton to my department head, and both of us were called into Whitehall—where the ministry reside—for an urgent meeting. While there we were told in no uncertain terms that the ministry opposed the book in its current form and would continue to do so in any form, even fictionalized. They worried the book might damage the interests of the United Kingdom internationally, seriously obstruct the promotion or protection by the United Kingdom of those interests, or endanger the safety of British citizens abroad. They suggested that any misconduct as reported in the manuscript could mean they might investigate these individuals. One of the deployed surgeons most likely to be at risk wrote to the surgeon general of his own accord, telling him that "there is nothing in the Bastion story that is made up" and expressing the "hope that the 'Bastion story' is accepted as a true representation of those six weeks, as I believe it is." I subsequently sent this surgeon a more developed version of the manuscript for his perusal, accommodated the few minor concerns he had, and accepted his blessing to proceed with publication.

In a separate letter, and after having delayed the matter for many months, the surgeon general expressed his concern that it would be "extremely difficult to provide a reader in a work of this nature with the necessary depth and background to understand complex clinical decision-making in a war zone. This may lead to excerpts being read out of context which is my principal concern regarding the publication of this manuscript." This is, I think, a fair concern, and I have done my best to fill in at least some of the background. The manuscript contains only a few examples of clinical decision making, and where they do exist they are described principally in terms of how these decisions were experienced by the doctors and nurses involved.

In his letter, the surgeon general also included a list of objections—something that I had asked for eighteen months earlier. This list, when it finally did arrive, contained fifty-five numbered objections organized along four categories: reputation, patient confidentiality, staff identification, and coalition/operational security. Perhaps unsurprisingly, of these objections, 90 percent related to concerns with the Ministry of Defence's reputation.

In fairness, my worry was never really with the legal implications of publication: I did what I did in good faith and without violating any signed agreement (which was easy enough to do, as I was never asked to sign any paperwork). I took care to disguise the identities of patients as best I could. Where people told me things in confidence—whether patients or staff—I always respected this confidence. A commissioned opinion, a "legal read," by a reputable London-based law firm that specializes in precisely this sort of thing, made it clear that the ministry had no legal basis on which to file an injunction against, or otherwise prohibit publication of the book, and reassured me that the MoD's bravado and bullying were entirely true to type.

What did bother me, and does still, are my moral obligations to those I deployed with. Not only do I genuinely respect what they do, but I have been concerned not to put them in harm's way by means of a straightforward, descriptive account of life in, and behind, the scenes in a war hospital, even if this is what they themselves wished for. To achieve that I did what I could to render the manuscript unreliable if it were ever used as evidence in a witch hunt, by obscuring identities and, in very rare cases, by means of deliberate misattribution. I also destroyed the hard drive that contained my original field notes.

That ethnography can, and often does, lead to feelings of betrayal is nothing new. To be on the receiving end of betrayal was, however, new to me. However noble the intentions, and however balanced an ethnography one seeks to write, it invariably risks being seen as biased, inaccurate, partial, and exploitative by those who provided the raw material in the first place. I was reminded of Bronisław Malinowski's controversial *A Diary in the Strict Sense of the Term*, a meticulous record of the time he spent observing natives. It revealed a quite different world from that described in his authoritative text on the Western Pacific. And it was this diary, said Clifford Geertz, that blew the straw house of ethnography to bits, leaving its author accused of doing the dirty on the discipline. As Geertz wrote subsequently, most of the shock arose from the discovery that Malinowski was not, to put it delicately, an unmitigated nice guy. He had rude things to say about the natives he was living with and rude words to say them in. He spent a great deal of time wishing he were elsewhere.

Similarly, Caroline Brettell wrote about the reception of Nancy Scheper-Hughes's work on the people of Ballybran:

> On the one hand were those who, like one Inis Beag woman, thought that "everything he . . . says is true." . . . Yet this woman commented to an Irish colleague . . . that the reason he would be lynched if he returned to Inis Beag was that "he had a right not to say it." Like the people of Ballybran and Springdale, the islanders were most offended by the fact that the private had become public—that the ethnographer had foregrounded what the people studied wish to maintain in the background.[3]

She quoted the village schoolmaster: "It's not your science I'm questioning, but this: don't we have the right to lead unexamined lives, the right not to be analysed? Don't we have a right to hold on to an image of ourselves as different to be sure, but as innocent and unblemished all the same?"[4] As Brettell pointed out, it was one thing to publish ethnographies about Trobrianders or Kwakiutls half a century ago; it is quite another to study people who read what you write and are more than willing to talk back.[5]

Journalism, of course, grapples with a similar issue. Andrew Sullivan, a columnist for the *Sunday Times*, is unequivocal on the matter: "The last thing a journalist needs to be is answerable for the consequences of his stories, as long as they are accurate and written in good faith. What a hack needs is to be relentless in pursuit of what the truth is—and to parlay that into a confection that readers want and enjoy and learn from."[6]

If only things were that straightforward in ethnography. Fieldwork requires us to spend extended periods of time reliant on the hospitality, and quite often the friendship, of our subjects. While some will be judicious and somewhat cautious, the best informants are not. They continue life as if we weren't there at all. As a matter of fact, the point of embedding for extended periods is partly that time will erode distinctions between observer and observed, creating the best possible conditions for natural behaviors to be displayed.

In Camp Bastion's field hospital, for the most part, I would like to think that these distinctions did erode. If this account has shown the doctors' lives to be a little messier than the hospital's accomplishments may have led one to expect, it might be our expectation that needs challenging. After all, what do we expect when placing people in situations where they see daily the tragic human consequence of war, and a very large amount of it? They brought to war, as we would too, all that made them human: their insecurities and competitive streaks, likes and dislikes, their expectations of self and others, their principles and charities, their want of family and friends, their hopes and their hang-ups. It is only because they are human that they can be heroes. For such qualities as courage and altruism are meaningless if not set against such human traits as self-doubt, and laziness, and the tendency to look after oneself first and foremost. This then is their story: a candid narrative that is admiring of the commitment and fearlessness of the doctors and nurses who, unlike you and me, have strong enough stomachs to mop up what we destroy.

By Way of Acknowledgment

This book, like so many, wouldn't exist if not for the encouragement and help of others. First and foremost, I'd like to thank those I deployed with (you know who you are). The camaraderie you provided was second to none, and I miss it still. There is something very special about the friendships that develop within the armed forces, and I was lucky to be given a taste of it. I especially value the comradeship of Anthony Lambert, a true one-of-a-kind, and generous to a fault. I also appreciate the support of Mark Midwinter and Pete Mahoney.

When the original manuscript ran into trouble, a number of people came to my help: Sandra Dawson, Christoph Loch, Tim Bellis, Stephanie Palmer, Lucy Moorman, Charhazad Abdullah, and Richard Hytner. Others provided invaluable inputs into structuring and editing the manuscript, occasionally against a tight deadline: John Van Maanen, Matthew Rothschild, Andrew Howard, Massey Beveridge, Florian Roessler, Marcus Georgio, Bud Goodall, Tom Scott, Frank Ledwidge, Jennifer Howard-Grenville, Jaco Lok, and Cornell's Suzanne Gordon, Ange Romeo-Hall, and Frances Benson. Dvora Yanow's collegiality and fine editing skills proved exceptionally helpful, and illustrative of the best that our scholarly community has to offer. Some gave more than others, and several gave far more than could have reasonably been expected. All did so without hesitation, and without reward. The book is far better for their input.

Last but certainly not least, there are those who provided moral support throughout, and none more so than my beautiful daughters Shelby and Dylan, and my partner Magda Rakita, a talented documentary photographer.

Notes

1. The ISAF alliance included NATO members: Albania, Belgium, Bulgaria, Canada, Croatia, the Czech Republic, Denmark, Estonia, France, Germany, Greece, Hungary, Iceland, Italy, Latvia, Lithuania, Luxembourg, the Netherlands, Norway, Poland, Portugal, Romania, Slovakia, Slovenia, Spain, Turkey, the United Kingdom, and the United States, as well as members of the Euro-Atlantic Partnership Council (EAPC): Armenia, Austria, Azerbaijan, Bosnia and Herzegovina, Finland, Georgia, Ireland, Macedonia, Montenegro, Sweden, Switzerland, Ukraine, and several non-NATO and non-EAPC countries: Australia, Bahrain, El Salvador, Jordan, Malaysia, Mongolia, New Zealand, Singapore, South Korea, Tonga, and the United Arab Emirates.

2. The British code name for the US-led Operation Enduring Freedom was Operation Herrick.

3. Source: Ministry of Defence, Defence Statistics Health, https://www.gov.uk/government/uploads/system/uploads/attachment_data/file/280507/recovery-rate-of-UK-service-personnel-admitted-to-camp-bastion-field-hospital.pdf.

4. Source: http://icasualties.org/oef/.

5. A report titled *Body Count* put together by Physicians for Social Responsibility, Physicians for Global Survival, and the Nobel Peace Prize–winning International Physicians for the Prevention of Nuclear War concluded that 106,000–170,000 civilians have been killed as a result of the fighting in Afghanistan at the hands of all parties to the conflict.

6. Source: UNICEF, 1986, as cited in Derek Summerfield, *The Impact of War and Atrocity on Civilian Populations: Basic Principles for NGO Interventions and a Critique of Psychosocial Trauma Projects* (London: Overseas Development Institute, 1996).

7. I returned to Afghanistan in December 2015 for a twelve-day exploratory study into the impact of war on civilians, funded by the British and Irish

Afghanistan Agencies Group. Despite high PTSD estimates (from 44 percent to 62 percent), neither the country's first-ever private neuropsychiatric hospital in Mazar-e-Sharif nor the city's civil hospital seems to use PTSD as a diagnosis. Patient records of a mental health clinic in Herat operated by International Assistance Mission suggested that only 1.2 percent were diagnosed with PTSD. The likely reason for this "absence" of PTSD is that depression and anxiety are usually quicker to diagnose, and consultations are typically "one-offs" and short in duration, especially because people usually have to travel far to get treatment. Moreover, PTSD often occurs in combination with depression and anxiety, so treating the latter pharmacologically (typically with a generic selective serotonin reuptake inhibitor) means a likely easing of symptoms in any event.

8. A tracheotomy is an incision in the windpipe made to relieve an obstruction to breathing. A fasciotomy is a surgical procedure where the fascia is cut to relieve tension or pressure, commonly to treat the resulting loss of circulation to an area of tissue or muscle; it is also a limb-saving procedure when used to treat acute compartment syndrome. A laparotomy is a surgical procedure involving a large incision through the abdominal wall to gain access to the abdominal cavity; it is also known as a celiotomy. A thoracotomy is an incision into the pleural space of the chest.

9. Damage-control resuscitation focuses on time-efficient surgery for victims with multiple or severe injuries and is usually used as an opposite of early definitive surgical management. Surgeries in Camp Bastion's field hospital were typically designed to control damage until definitive surgery could take place (usually back in the UK or the United States, or in an Afghan hospital). Thus, these damage-control surgeries would often leave packs in the abdomen (to stop internal bleeding) or place temporary fixation for fractures (often using external fixators).

10. Tim Kreider, "The Power of 'I Don't Know,'" *New York Times*, April 29, 2013, http://opinionator.blogs.nytimes.com/2013/04/29/the-power-of-i-dont-know/?_r=0.

11. Kurt Vonnegut, *Slaughterhouse-Five* (London: Vintage Classics, 1991).

1. Hawkeye

1. All names used in this book are pseudonyms. The name "Hawkeye" has been adopted from Richard Hooker's protagonist in *MASH*, as the general surgeon in question bore an uncanny resemblance to Hooker's fictional character Benjamin Franklin "Hawkeye" Pierce.

2. Reporting for Duty

1. Ernest Becker, *The Denial of Death* (London: Souvenir Press, 1973), 282–83.

2. H. S. Becker, B. Geer, E. C. Hughes, and A. L. Strauss, *Boys in White: Student Culture in Medical School* (Chicago: University of Chicago Press, 1961). See also L. D. Henman, "Humor as a Coping Mechanism: Lessons from POWs," *Humor* 14, no. 1 (2001): 83–94.

3. D. Wear, J. M. Aultman, J. D. Varley, and J. Zarconi, "Making Fun of Patients: Medical Students' Perceptions and Use of Derogatory and Cynical Humor in Clinical Settings," *Academic Medicine* 81, no. 5 (2006): 454–62.

4. Excerpt from Howard Jacobson, *Zoo Time* (London: Bloomsbury, 2012), 279.

5. Attributed to Leon Bloy.

3. Camp Bastion

1. Patrick Wintour, "Bleak Camp Bastion—and a Vision of Roses and Saffron," *Guardian*, November 21, 2006.

4. A Reason to Live

1. Excerpt from Stephen Wright, *Meditations in Green* (London: Penguin, Sphere, 1987), 196.

2. See Frank Ledwidge, *Losing Small Wars: British Military Failure in Iraq and Afghanistan* (London: Yale University Press, 2011), 71. Also, a recent, and fairly controversial, *New York Times* article relied on court records and interviews to explore the psychological damage suffered by American soldiers told not to intervene (not even when the abuse took place on American bases), as this was considered a matter for domestic Afghan criminal law; see http://www.nytimes.com/2015/09/21/world/asia/us-soldiers-told-to-ignore-afghan-allies-abuse-of-boys.html?_r=0.

3. Ben Anderson's "This Is What Winning Looks Like" can be viewed on http://www.informationclearinghouse.info/article37216.htm.

4. Excerpt from Richard Hooker, *MASH* (London: Sphere, 1973), 111.

5. For a more extensive treatment of psychological injury at war, see M. de Rond and J. Lok, "Some Things Can Never Be Unseen: The Role of Context in Psychological Injury at War," *Academy of Management Journal* (forthcoming), from which this piece of text was adapted.

6. Apocalypse Now and Again

1. Michael Herr, *Dispatches* (London: Picador, 1977), 207.

2. Quoted in Frank Ledwidge, *Losing Small Wars: British Military Failure in Iraq and Afghanistan* (London: Yale University Press, 2011), 198.

3. Anthony Loyd, *My War Gone By, I Miss It So* (London: Anchor, 2000), 168.

4. From William James, *The Will to Believe* (1896; London: Dover, 2003), 31.

5. I owe this expression (although I paraphrase) to Graham Greene, *The Burnt-Out Case* (Kingswood, UK: Windmill, 1961), 247.

6. Attributed to International Committee of the Red Cross (ICRC) founder Jean-Henri Dunant, and as cited in Michael Ignatieff, *The Warrior's Honor: Ethnic War and the Modern Conscience* (New York: Holt, 1998), 110.

7. Marco Giannangeli, "Desperate Soldiers Self-Harm in Bid to Escape Afghanistan," *Express*, http://www.express.co.uk/posts/view/356011/Desperate-soldiers-self-harm-in-bid-to-escape-Afghanistan.

8. From Rudyard Kipling, "The Young British Soldier," quoted in Ledwidge, *Losing Small Wars*, 61.

7. Boredom

1. Constructive criticism during weekly case reviews is a normal and positive part of medical practice. It is not uncommon for these exercises to cross well past the line of a collegial discussion and enter into a blame game or involve posturing, particularly where strong personalities are involved or cases are ambiguous and high stakes. Seasoned surgeons are relatively thick-skinned, but junior doctors in particular can feel intimidated and will not often open up about that aspect of their experience. This sentence unpacks into all kinds of important ethnographic questions.

2. Excerpt from Stephen Wright, *Meditations in Green* (London: Penguin, Sphere, 1987), 23.

3. Excerpt from Norman Mailer, *The Naked and the Dead* (New York: Rinehart & Co., 1949), 8–9.

4. A US marine (Steiner) quoted in Tim Hetherington, *Infidel* (London: Chris Boot, 2010), 193.

5. A US marine (O'Byrne) quoted ibid., 109.

6. Ibid., 15.

7. Don McCullin, *Unreasonable Behaviour* (London: Vintage, 2002), 100–101.

8. Christmas in Summer

1. Excerpt from Phil Clay, "Redeployment," in *The Best American Nonrequired Reading* (New York: Houghton, Mifflin, Harcourt, 2012), 119; originally published in *Granta*.

2. Morbidity and mortality (M&M) meetings are traditional, recurring conferences held by medical services at academic medical centers, most large private medical and surgical practices, and other medical centers. They are usually peer reviews of mistakes occurring during the care of patients.

3. Complications like this are common despite the best attempt to do the right thing at the time. Good morbidity and mortality reviews focus on what is system preventable rather than people preventable, for instance by stocking pediatric-size tubes and needles in the air evacuation equipment.

4. Peter L. Berger and Thomas Luckmann, *The Social Construction of Reality: A Treatise in the Sociology of Knowledge* (London: Penguin, 1991).

10. Kandahar

1. Camp "Atul" Hero is a corps-level formation of the Afghan National Army and includes a regional hospital. It is located in Kandahar, adjacent to Kandahar Airfield.

2. This description is not all that far removed from the sociologist Erving Goffman's definition of "total institutions" in his *Asylums: Essays on the Social Situations of Mental Patients and Other Inmates* (London: Penguin, 1991).

11. War Is Nasty

1. During surgical procedures, scrub nurses typically assist the surgeon by organizing and passing equipment and supplies (instruments, sponges, sutures). Occasionally, scrub nurses will assist more directly, for instance by holding a retractor to allow the surgeon a better view inside a cavity, or by working the suction or electrocautery machine. If there are enough doctors as assistants, the scrub nurse may never need to take on such tasks, which are an integral part of the operative procedure. Surgeons can be very defensive of their scrub nurses, as they rely so heavily on them.

2. Ernest Becker, *The Denial of Death* (London: Souvenir, 1973), xii.

3. Eric Hobsbawm, "War and Peace," *Guardian*, February 22, 2002, http://www.theguardian.com/education/2002/feb/23/artsandhumanities.highereducation.

4. Source: *Analysis of VA Health Care Utilization among Operation Enduring Freedom (OEF), Operation Iraqi Freedom (OIF), and Operation New Dawn (OND) Veterans*, US Department of Veterans Affairs, http://www.publichealth.va.gov/docs/epidemiology/healthcare-utilization-report-fy2014-qtr4.pdf.

5. Source: Dave Baiocchi, "Measuring Army Deployments to Iraq and Afghanistan," Rand Corporation, 2013, http://www.rand.org/content/dam/rand/pubs/research_reports/RR100/RR145/RAND_RR145.pdf.

6. Source: "PTSD in Service Members and New Veterans of the Iraq and Afghanistan Wars: A Bibliography and Critique," *PTSD Research Quarterly* 20, no. 1 (2009), http://www.ptsd.va.gov/professional/newsletters/research-quarterly/V20N1.pdf.

7. According to a study published in the *Lancet*, 650,000 had already died in Iraq alone by 2004 (see http://web.mit.edu/humancostiraq/).

8. Source: "Darfur Conflict," *Thompson Reuters Foundation News*, updated July 31, 2014, http://www.trust.org/spotlight/Darfur-conflict.

9. Source: "Combat Stress Sees Fourfold Increase in Veterans Seeking Help for Mental Health," Combat Stress, December 7, 2015, http://www.combatstress.org.uk/news/2015/12/20-year-referral-paper/.

10. N. Greenberg, E. Jones, N. Jones, N. T. Fear, and S. Wessely, "The Injured Mind in the UK Armed Forces," *Philosophical Transactions of the Royal Society B* 366 (2011): 261–67.

11. Ibid.

12. N. T. Fear, M. Jones, D. Murphy, L. Hull, A. C. Iversen, B. Coker, L. Machell, et al., "What Are the Consequences of Deployment to Iraq and Afghanistan on the Mental Health of the UK Armed Forces? A Cohort Study," *Lancet* 375, no. 9728 (2010): 1783–97. See also A. C. Iversen and N. Greenberg, "Mental Health of Regular and Reserve Military Veterans," *Advances in Psychiatric Treatment* 15, no. 2 (2009): 100–106. And I. G. Jacobson, M. A. Ryan, T. I. Hooper, T. C. Smith, P. J. Amoroso, E. J. Boyko, G. D. Gackstetter, T. S. Wells, and N. S. Bell, "Alcohol Use and Alcohol-Related Problems before and after Military Combat Deployment," *Journal of the American Medical Association* 300, no. 6 (2008): 663–75.

13. For an explanation of the differences between ICD-10 and DSM-5 see US Department of Veterans Affairs, "PTSD: National Center for PTSD," http://www.ptsd.va.gov/professional/assessment/overview/comparison-icd-dsm-iv.asp.

14. D. MacManus, N. Jones, S. Wessely, N. T. Fear, E. Jones, and N. Greenberg, "The Mental Health of the UK Armed Forces in the 21st Century: Resilience in the Face of Adversity," *Journal of the Royal Army Medical Corps* 160 (2014): 125–30, doi:10.1136/jramc-2013-000213.

15. J. Firth-Cozens, S. J. Midgley, and C. Burges, "Questionnaire Survey of Post-traumatic Stress Disorder in Doctors Involved in the Omagh Bombing," *British Medical Journal* 319, no. 7225 (1999): 1609. See also A. Weinberg and F. Creed, "Stress and Psychiatric Disorder in Healthcare Professionals and Hospital Staff," *Lancet* 355, no. 9203 (2000): 533–37. And see Y. Palgi, M. Ben-Ezra, S. Langer, and N. Essar, "The Effect of Prolonged Exposure to War Stress on the Comorbidity of PTSD and Depression among Hospital Personnel," *Psychiatry Research* 168, no. 3 (2009): 262–64.

16. M. Jones, N. T. Fear, N. Greenberg, N. Jones, L. Hull, M. Hotopf, S. Wessely, and R. J. Rona, "Do Medical Services Personnel Who Deployed to the Iraq War Have Worse Mental Health Than Other Deployed Personnel?," *European Journal of Public Health* 18, no. 4 (2008): 422–27.

17. P. Cawkill, M. Jones, N. T. Fear, M. Fertout, S. Wessely, and N. Greenberg, "Mental Health of UK Armed Forces Medical Personnel Post-deployment," *Occupational Medicine* 65 (2015): 157–64.

18. M. Jones et al., "Do Medical Services Personnel Who Deployed to the Iraq War Have Worse Mental Health?," 422–27.

19. S. L. Hatch, S. B. Harvey, C. Dandeker, H. Burdett, N. Greenberg, N. T. Fear, and S. Wesseley, "Life in and after the Armed Forces: Social Networks and Mental Health in the UK Military," *Sociology of Health & Illness* 35, no. 7 (2013): 1045–64. See also M. Hotopf, L. Hull, N. T. Fear, T. Browne, O. Horn, A. Iversen, M. Jones, et al., "The Health of UK Military Personnel Who Deployed to the 2003 Iraq War: A Cohort Study," *Lancet* 367, no. 9524 (2006): 1731–41.

20. M.J. Friedman, "Post Traumatic Stress Disorder among Military Returnees from Afghanistan and Iraq," *American Journal of Psychiatry* 163, no. 4 (2006): 586–93. See also L.I. Pearlin and C. Schooler, "Structure of Coping," *Journal of Health and Social Behavior* 19, no. 1 (1978): 2–21; and L.I. Pearlin and C. Schooler, "Some Extensions of the Structure of Coping," *Journal of Health and Social Behavior* 20, no. 2 (1979): 202–5. And see M. Zeidner and N. S. Endler, *Handbook of Coping: Theory, Research, Applications* (London: Wiley, 1995).

21. Chris Hedges, *War Is a Force That Gives Us Meaning* (New York: Anchor Books), 3.

22. S.M. Lyman and M. B. Scott, *A Sociology of the Absurd* (New York: Appleton-Century-Crofts, 1970).

23. G.S. Arul, S. Bree, B. Sonka, C. Edwards, and P. Reavley, "The Secret Lives of the Bastion Bakers," *British Medical Journal* 349 (December 2014): 15–17, doi: http://dx.doi.org/10.1136/bmj.g7448.

24. For a more extensive treatment of psychological injury at war, see M. de Rond and J. Lok, "Some Things Can Never Be Unseen: The Role of Context in Psychological Injury at War," *Academy of Management Journal* (forthcoming), from which this piece of text was adapted.

12. Way to Start Your Day

1. Excerpt from Richard Hooker, *MASH* (London: Sphere, 1973), 21.

13. Back Home

1. I am aware that these two concluding paragraphs are similar to what I originally wrote in an essay for a journal. What I felt then, I still feel today, and my convictions remain unchanged. The essay in question is: M. de Rond, "Soldier, Surgeon, Photographer, Fly: Fieldwork beyond the Comfort Zone," *Strategic Organization* 10, no. 3 (2012): 256.

2. Edmund Burke, *A Philosophical Enquiry into the Origin of Our Ideas of the Sublime and Beautiful* (1757), as quoted in Susan Sontag, *Regarding the Pain of Others* (London: Penguin, 2003), 87.

3. Dave Grossman, *On Killing: The Psychological Cost of Learning to Kill in War and Society* (New York: Little, Brown, 2009), 236–37.

4. Ernest Hemingway, "On the Blue Water," *Esquire*, April 1936.

5. Tim Hetherington, *Infidel* (London: Chris Boot, 2010), 189–90.

6. The quote is from John Steinbeck, *Journal of a Novel: The East of Eden Letters* (New York: Viking, 1969), March 28, 1951, entry.

7. Lillian Smith, *Killers of the Dream* (New York: W. W. Norton, 1994).

Epilogue

1. A DA Notice is an official request to news editors not to publish or broadcast items on specified subjects for reasons of national security. The system is still in use in the United Kingdom.

2. Toby Harnden, "Pulped by the MoD," *Spectator*, March 12, 2011, http://www.spectator.co.uk/features/6766648/pulped-by-the-mod/.

3. Quoted in Caroline Brettell, *When They Read What We Write: The Politics of Ethnography* (Westport, CT: Bergin & Garvey, 1996), 14.

4. Quoted ibid., 13.

5. Caroline Brettell is quoting Paredes (1978).

6. Andrew Sullivan, *Sunday Times*, July 29, 2012, News Review, 4.